T0226832

Tickborne Borrelia Infections

Editor

ELITZA S. THEEL

CLINICS IN LABORATORY MEDICINE

www.labmed.theclinics.com

December 2015 • Volume 35 • Number 4

ELSEVIER

1600 John F. Kennedy Boulevard • Suite 1800 • Philadelphia, Pennsylvania, 19103-2899

http://www.theclinics.com

CLINICS IN LABORATORY MEDICINE Volume 35, Number 4
December 2015 ISSN 0272-2712, ISBN-13: 978-0-323-40254-5

Editor: Lauren Boyle
Developmental Editor: Colleen Viola

Reprints. For copies of 100 or more, of articles in this publication, please contact the Commercial Reprints Department, Elsevier Inc., 360 Park Avenue South, New York, New York 10010-1710. Tel. 212-633-3874, Fax: 212-633-3820, E-mail: reprints@elsevier.com.

Clinics in Laboratory Medicine (ISSN 0272-2712) is published quarterly by Elsevier Inc., 360 Park Avenue South, New York, NY 10010-1710. Months of issue are March, June, September, and December. Business and Editorial offices: 1600 John F. Kennedy Blvd., Suite 1800, Philadelphia, PA 19103-2899. Periodicals postage paid at NewYork, NY and additional mailing offices. Subscription prices are $250.00 per year (US individuals), $419.00 per year (US institutions), $135.00 per year (US students), $305.00 per year (Canadian individuals), $510.00 per year (Canadian institutions), $185.00 per year (Canadian students), $390.00 per year (international individuals), $510.00 per year (international institutions), $185.00 (international students). Foreign air speed delivery is included in all Clinics subscription prices. All prices are subject to change without notice. POSTMASTER: Send address changes to *Clinics in Laboratory Medicine,* Elsevier Health Sciences Division, Subscription Customer Service, 3251 Riverport Lane, Maryland Heights, MO 63043. **Customer Service: 1-800-654-2452 (US). From outside of the US and Canada, call 1-314-447-8871. Fax: 1-314-447-8029. E-mail: journalscustomerservice-usa@elsevier.com (for print support) or journalsonlinesupport-usa@elsevier.com (for online support).**

Clinics in Laboratory Medicine is covered in *EMBASE/Exerpta Medica, MEDLINE/PubMed (Index Medicus), Cinahl, Current Contents/Clinical Medicine, BIOSIS* and *ISI/BIOMED.*

Contributors

EDITOR

ELITZA S. THEEL, PhD, D(ABMM)
Assistant Professor, Department of Laboratory Medicine and Pathology, Mayo Clinic, Rochester, Minnesota

AUTHORS

KEVIN ALBY, PhD, D(ABMM)
Assistant Director, Clinical Microbiology; Assistant Professor, Department of Pathology and Laboratory Medicine, Perelman School of Medicine, University of Pennsylvania, Philadelphia, Pennsylvania

VICTOR P. BERARDI
Associate Director for Laboratory Science and CEO, Imugen, Inc, Norwood, Massachusetts

GERALD A. CAPRARO, PhD, D(ABMM)
Medical Director, Clinical Microbiology and Diagnostic Virology Laboratories; Assistant Professor, Department of Pathology and Translational Pathobiology, Louisiana State University Health Sciences Center – Shreveport, Shreveport, Louisiana

ADAM J. CAULFIELD, PhD
Instructor, Division of Clinical Microbiology, Department of Laboratory Medicine and Pathology, Mayo Clinic, Rochester, Minnesota

HANUMARA RAM CHOWDRI, MD
Hawthorn Medical Associates, New Bedford, Massachusetts

SALLY J. CUTLER, PhD
Professor in Medical Microbiology, School of Health, Sport and Bioscience, University of East London, London, United Kingdom

HOLLY M. FROST, MD
Department of Pediatrics, Marshfield Clinic, Minocqua, Wisconsin

HEIDI K. GOETHERT, ScD
Research Associate, Department of Infectious Disease and Global Health, Tufts University, Cummings School of Veterinary Medicine, North Grafton, Massachusetts

JOSEPH L. GUGLIOTTA, MD
Hunterdon Medical Center Infectious Diseases, Flemington, New Jersey

JOHN J. HALPERIN, MD
Chair, Department of Neurosciences, Overlook Medical Center, Summit, New Jersey; Professor of Neurology and Medicine, Sidney Kimmel Medical College of Thomas Jefferson University, Philadelphia, Pennsylvania

TIMOTHY J. LEPORE, MD
Nantucket Cottage Hospital, Nantucket, Massachusetts

L. ROBBIN LINDSAY, PhD
Research Scientist, National Microbiology Laboratory, Public Health Agency of Canada, Winnipeg, Manitoba, Canada

PHILIP J. MOLLOY, MD
Medical Director, Imugen, Inc, Norwood, Massachusetts

NICK H. OGDEN, DPhil
Senior Research Scientist, National Microbiology Laboratory, Public Health Agency of Canada, Saint-Hyacinthe, Quebec, Canada

MARY PETZKE, PhD
Department of Microbiology and Immunology, New York Medical College, Valhalla, New York

BOBBI S. PRITT, MD, MSc
Associate Professor, Division of Clinical Microbiology, Department of Laboratory Medicine and Pathology, Mayo Clinic, Rochester, Minnesota

JOYCE L. SANCHEZ, MD
Assistant Professor of Medicine, Divisions of General Internal Medicine and Infectious Diseases, Mayo Clinic, Rochester, Minnesota

STEVEN W. SCHOFIELD, PhD
Senior Advisor, Communicable Disease Control Program, Force Health Protection, Department of National Defence, Ottawa, Ontario, Canada

ANNA M. SCHOTTHOEFER, PhD
Marshfield Clinic Research Foundation, Marshfield, Wisconsin

MARTIN E. SCHRIEFER, PhD
Bacterial Disease Branch, Division of Vector-Borne Disease, Centers for Disease Control and Prevention, Fort Collins, Colorado

IRA SCHWARTZ, PhD
Department of Microbiology and Immunology, New York Medical College, Valhalla, New York

SAM R. TELFORD III, ScD
Professor, Department of Infectious Disease and Global Health, Tufts University, Cummings School of Veterinary Medicine, North Grafton, Massachusetts

Contents

Lyme borreliosis is a zoonotic, tick-borne disease that infects humans worldwide. The disease is currently recognized as the most common vector-borne disease in Europe and North America. Disease is caused by several genospecies of the *Borrelia burgdorferi* sensu lato complex. Humans are at high risk of infection in regions where highly competent reservoirs are the primary hosts for the subadult stages of the tick, in contrast to regions where less competent or refractory animals feed ticks. Human infections are also most frequently associated with spring and summer months when the nymph stage of the tick is active.

Borrelia burgdorferi is the tick-borne etiologic agent of Lyme disease. The spirochete must negotiate numerous barriers in order to establish a disseminated infection in a mammalian host. These barriers include migration from the feeding tick midgut to the salivary glands, deposition in skin, manipulation or evasion of the localized host immune response, adhesion to and extravasation through an endothelial barrier, hematogenous dissemination, and establishment of infection in distal tissue sites. *Borrelia burgdorferi* proteins that mediate many of these processes and the nature of the host response to infection are described.

Lyme disease is the most common tick-borne illness in the United States and is also seen in areas of Europe and Asia. The growing deer and *Ixodes* species tick populations in many areas underscore the importance of clinicians to properly recognize and treat the different stages of Lyme disease. Controversy regarding the cause and management of persistent symptoms following treatment of Lyme disease persists and is highlighted in this review.

Nervous system involvement occurs in 10% to 15% of patients infected with the tick-borne spirochetes *Borrelia burgdorferi*, *B afzelii*, and *B garinii*. Peripheral nervous system involvement is common. Central nervous system (CNS) involvement, most commonly presenting with lymphocytic meningitis, causes modest cerebrospinal fluid (CSF) pleocytosis. Parenchymal CNS infection is rare. If the CNS is invaded, however, measuring local production of anti– *B burgdorferi* antibodies in the CSF provides a useful marker of infection. Most cases of neuroborreliosis can be cured with oral doxycycline; parenteral regimens should be reserved for patients with particularly severe disease.

Serology is the mainstay of confirmation of Lyme borreliosis; direct detection has limited application. Because standardized 2-tier testing (STTT) has been commonly used since the mid 1990s, standardization and performance have improved. STTT detection of early, localized infection is poor; that of late disease is good. The best indicator of stage 1 infection, erythema migrans, is presented in the majority of US cases and should prompt treatment without testing. Clinical and epidemiologic correlates should be carefully assessed before ordering STTT. STTT has great value in confirming extracutaneous infection. Recent developments promise to improve performance, particularly in early disease detection.

Although serologic testing remains the gold standard for laboratory diagnosis of Lyme disease, the antibody response may take several weeks to increase greater than the limit of detection. Because of this extended time frame, it is necessary to identify new diagnostic methods for earlier diagnosis and appropriate treatment of Lyme disease. Alternative diagnostic modalities, such as *Borrelia* culture or nucleic acid amplification testing, may be beneficial in specific clinical scenarios. In early phases of acute infection, before the development of an immune response, detection of *Borrelia* DNA from clinical specimens may help establish the diagnosis sooner than serologic methods.

Lyme disease in North America is caused by infection with the spirochetal bacterium *Borrelia burgdorferi* and transmitted by *Ixodes scapularis* and *Ixodes pacificus* ticks. These ticks also have the potential to transmit a rapidly expanding list of other pathogenic bacteria, viruses, and parasites, including *Anaplasma phagocytophilum*, *Babesia microti*, deer tick (Powassan) virus, *Borrelia miyamotoi*, and the *Ehrlichia muris*–like organism. Coinfections with *B burgdorferi* and these other agents are often difficult to diagnose and may go untreated, and thus contribute significantly to patient morbidity and mortality from tick-borne infections.

Sally J. Cutler

Relapsing fever borreliae were notorious and feared infectious agents that earned their place in history through their devastating impact as causes of both epidemic and endemic infection. They are now considered more as an oddity, and their burden of infection is largely overshadowed by other infections such as malaria, which presents in a similar clinical way. Despite this, they remain the most common bacterial infection in some developing countries. Transmitted by soft ticks or lice, these fascinating spirochetes have evolved a myriad of mechanisms to survive within their diverse environments.

Sam R. Telford III, Heidi K. Goethert, Philip J. Molloy, Victor P. Berardi, Hanumara Ram Chowdri, Joseph L. Gugliotta, and Timothy J. Lepore

Borrelia miyamotoi disease (BMD) is a newly recognized borreliosis globally transmitted by ticks of the *Ixodes persulcatus* species complex. Once considered to be a tick symbiont with no public health implications, *B miyamotoi* is increasingly recognized as the agent of a nonspecific febrile illness often misdiagnosed as acute Lyme disease without rash, or as ehrlichiosis. The frequency of its diagnosis in the northeastern United States is similar to that of human granulocytic ehrlichiosis. A diagnosis of BMD is confirmed by polymerase chain reaction analysis of acute blood samples, or by seroconversion using a recombinant glycerophosphodiester phosphodiesterase enzyme immunoassay. BMD is successfully treated with oral doxycycline or amoxicillin.

Nick H. Ogden, L. Robbin Lindsay, and Steven W. Schofield

Current approaches for prevention of tick bites, Lyme disease, and other tick-borne diseases are described. Particular attention is paid to 4 risk-reduction strategies: (i) avoiding risk areas; (ii) personal protective measures that reduce the risk of tick bites or transmission of the agent of Lyme disease, *Borrelia burgdorferi*; (iii) reducing the number of infected ticks in the environment; and (iv) use of prophylactic antibiotic treatments following a bite to prevent clinical Lyme disease.

CLINICS IN LABORATORY MEDICINE

THE CLINICS ARE NOW AVAILABLE ONLINE!
Access your subscription at:
www.theclinics.com

Preface

Tickborne *Borrelia* Infections: Beyond Just Lyme Disease

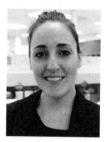

Elitza S. Theel, PhD, D(ABMM)
Editor

Members of the *Borrelia* genus are associated with two main clinical syndromes: Lyme borreliosis and relapsing fever. With a few exceptions, these spirochetes share many similarities, including transmission via blood feeding arthropods, environmental maintenance among rodent populations, and interruption of the lifecycle following human infection. As a result of the high annual incidence of Lyme disease in both the United States (approximately 300,000 cases) and Europe (approximately 85,000 cases from 18 countries), Lyme borreliosis and its causative agents (primarily *Borrelia burgdorferi* in the United States and *Borrelia afzelii* and *Borrelia garinii* in Europe) often garner the most attention from both the medical community and public forums. Relapsing fever *Borrelia* infections remain uncommon in the United States, with approximately 480 cases reported to the Centers for Disease Control and Prevention between 1990 and 2011. However, these numbers may be an underrepresentation of the true incidence of infection due to the lack of sensitive diagnostic tools to identify these agents and possibly clinician unfamiliarity with the medical entity. Relapsing fever, particularly tickborne relapsing fever, remains endemic in certain impoverished regions of the world, including East Africa, and thus the potential for spread or encountering these organisms in returning travelers or immigrants continues to exist. Finally, new species within the *Borrelia* genus continue to be identified, and most recently, this includes detailed characterization of *Borrelia miyamotoi*. While genetically closely related to relapsing fever borreliae, infection with *B miyamotoi* does not present with classic relapsing fever symptoms, but rather more closely resembles that of Lyme disease, though notably without a characteristic rash.

In this issue of *Clinics in Laboratory Medicine*, we delve into key aspects of Lyme disease, including an update on the epidemiology and the increasing geographic spread of *B burgdorferi* in the United States. In addition, a review of *B burgdorferi* pathogenesis and the associated host response is provided. The common and uncommon clinical manifestations of Lyme disease, with an in-depth discussion of Lyme neuroborreliosis,

Clin Lab Med 35 (2015) ix–x
http://dx.doi.org/10.1016/j.cll.2015.09.001
0272-2712/15/$ – see front matter © 2015 Published by Elsevier Inc.

labmed.theclinics.com

are presented, alongside a review of the consensus treatment guidelines. While the focus of this issue is on tickborne *Borrelia* infections, it is prudent to emphasize the risk of other tickborne infections that may be transmitted alongside *B burgdorferi*. Therefore, these potential coinfecting agents, including *Anaplasma phagocytophilum, Babesia microti,* Powassan (deer tick) virus, and others, are also reviewed. As serologic testing for Lyme disease remains the preferred diagnostic modality, the most recent advancements in this field are summarized, as are alternative methods of identification, including molecular testing and antigen detection. A detailed discussion of the relapsing fever borreliae and *B miyamotoi*, including their clinical presentation, diagnostic tools, and treatment options, is also provided. Finally, this issue concludes with an in-depth review of measures that can be taken to prevent tickborne infections, including available physical barriers and the status of vaccine development.

I would like to thank all of the authors for providing their expertise and time to make this yet another informative and exciting issue of the *Clinics in Laboratory Medicine* series. I would also like to thank Alexander McAdam, MD, PhD for initial guidance and discussion regarding the content of this issue and the Elsevier staff, especially Joanne Husovski and Colleen Viola, for their help throughout the process.

Elitza S. Theel, PhD, D(ABMM)
Department of Laboratory Medicine
and Pathology
Mayo Clinic
3050 Superior Drive, NW, Room 526
Rochester, MN 55901, USA

E-mail address:
theel.elitza@mayo.edu

Ecology and Epidemiology of Lyme Borreliosis

Anna M. Schotthoefer, PhD[a],*, Holly M. Frost, MD[b]

KEYWORDS

- Lyme disease • Borreliosis • *Borrelia burgdorferi* • Ecology • Epidemiology
- Incidence • *Ixodes*

KEY POINTS

- Current estimates suggest as many as 300,000 people in the United States and at least 85,000 people in Europe are infected with Lyme borreliosis each year, with evidence that prevalence of the disease is expanding worldwide.
- Most cases in the United States are caused by *Borrelia burgdorferi* sensu stricto, whereas *Borrelia afzelii* and *Borrelia garinii* cause most disease in Europe, although genetic studies are also revealing previously unrecognized pathogenic members of the *B burgdorferi* species complex.
- Many vertebrate species may be involved in the maintenance of the pathogen in nature. Small mammals, such as mice and shrews, may be particularly important reservoir hosts. Deer and birds may play important roles in the spread of tick populations and the geographic expansion of the disease.
- Genetic studies have allowed for the differentiation of strains that vary in their abilities to disseminate and cause chronic manifestations of Lyme disease, and which tend to be maintained in nature by different reservoir hosts.

INTRODUCTION

Lyme disease, also known as Lyme borreliosis, is caused by a complex of spirochete bacteria known collectively as *Borrelia burgdorferi* sensu lato (s.l.). The disease was first described in the 1970s in association with an epidemic of arthritis in young children in Old Lyme, Connecticut, USA.[1,2] Today, Lyme disease is the most common vector-borne disease in the Northern Hemisphere.[3] About 30,000 cases are reported annually to the Centers for Disease Control and Prevention (CDC) in the United States,[4] although a recent estimate suggested that as many as 300,000 people are

The authors have no disclosures to announce.
[a] Marshfield Clinic Research Foundation, 1000 North Oak Avenue, Marshfield, WI 54449, USA;
[b] Department of Pediatrics, Marshfield Clinic, 9601 Townline Road, Minocqua, WI 54548, USA
* Corresponding author.
E-mail address: Schotthoefer.Anna@mcrf.mfldclin.edu

Clin Lab Med 35 (2015) 723–743
http://dx.doi.org/10.1016/j.cll.2015.08.003

diagnosed each year with Lyme disease such that the actual number of people infected may be substantially higher.[5] Infections in Europe are also widespread. The World Health Organization estimated that more than 85,000 cases occur annually in Europe,[3] although the lack of a uniform reporting system makes tracking cases difficult.[6] Globally, Lyme disease has been reported in more than 80 countries, and it appears to be on the rise.[3,7]

The disease is complex, varying in its clinical presentation, and can at times be challenging to be reliably diagnosed using standard diagnostic tests, as discussed elsewhere in this issue. The life cycle of the pathogen and the ecological interactions that influence the risks of transmission to humans are also extremely complex, but are nonetheless important to understand in guiding the diagnosis, treatment, and control of the disease. In this review, the ecological aspects of Lyme disease, what is known about the pathogen, the vector, and the reservoir hosts across the Northern Hemisphere, and some of the factors that contribute to the transmission to humans are focused on.

GEOGRAPHIC DISTRIBUTION OF THE DISEASE

There are 2 main regions of high incidence in the United States, one occurring in the northeastern and mid-Atlantic states and the other in the upper Midwestern states. More than 90% of cases in the United States are reported from 14 states in these regions (**Fig. 1**).[4,8] In 2013, Vermont, New Hampshire, and Maine reported the highest incidence rates, ranging from around 80 to 100 cases per 100,000 people. Minnesota and Wisconsin in the upper Midwest reported incidence rates of about 25 per 100,000.[4] An additional endemic area occurs along the Pacific Coast in California, Oregon, and Washington (see **Fig. 1**).

Lyme borreliosis is found throughout Europe, Russia, and Asia. The highest reported frequencies of the disease are in central Europe and Scandinavia, particularly in Germany, Austria, Slovenia, the Baltic coastline of Sweden, and some Estonian and Finnish islands, where reported incidence rates are greater than 100 cases per 100,000.[3,9] Seroprevalence studies conducted in individual countries in recent years, including Germany, Denmark, and Sweden, have typically found positive rates less than 10%, although rates as high as 47.9% were recorded in high-risk groups (eg, farmers and forestry workers) in Poland.[3,10–13]

Globally, the incidence of Lyme disease is growing. In the United States, the number of confirmed cases of Lyme disease reported between 1995 and 2013 increased by about 130% from 11,700 to 27,203.[14] In Canada, the number of reported cases increased by nearly 8 times between 2004 and 2012,[15] and several studies in Europe have indicated similar increases.[3,16,17] This increase is secondary to a variety of influences including climate change resulting in the expansion of the *Ixodes* tick territory including expansion to higher elevations, changes in small mammal and deer populations, changes in deforestation and development, and improved reporting and awareness of disease.[3,8,18–21] Some studies have suggested increased *B burgdorferi* virulence may be contributing to global spread; however, studies looking at *B burgdorferi* populations in the United States have been unable to validate this.[21,22]

THE ETIOLOGIC AGENT

Lyme borreliosis is predominantly caused by 3 genospecies of the *B burgdorferi* sensu lato complex, *B burgdorferi* sensu stricto (hereafter referred to as *B burgdorferi*), *Borrelia afzelii*, and *Borrelia garinii*.[23,24] *B afzelii* and *B garinii* are the predominant organisms responsible for Lyme disease in Europe and Asia, although *B burgdorferi* may

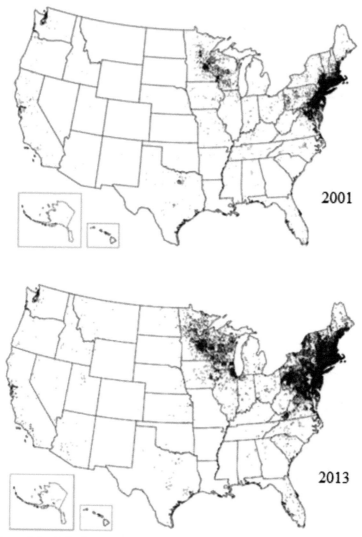

Fig. 1. Maps of the United States showing the concentration of reported cases of Lyme disease in the northeastern, mid-Atlantic, and upper Midwestern regions of the country. An increase in the number of reported cases and the expansion from these main focal regions is evident between 2001 and 2013. One dot represents one reported case. (*From* Lyme Disease. Centers for Disease Control and Prevention. Available at: http://www.cdc.gov/lyme/stats/index.html. Accessed September 9, 2015.)

also infect humans in those locations.[24–27] In North America, *B burgdorferi* was thought to be the only genospecies to cause Lyme disease[3,24,25]; however, new evidence uncovered by molecular analyses has suggested that disease there may also be caused by other sensu lato species.[28,29] At least 18 genospecies have been identified worldwide, some of which have been shown to have pathogenic potential in humans (**Table 1**).[25,30,31]

Table 1
Currently recognized members of the *Borrelia burgdorferi* sensu lato complex and what is known about their pathogenicity and life cycles

B burgdorferi sensu lato Species	Pathogenic to Humans?	Geographic Distribution	Vectors	Primary Reservoirs
B burgdorferi sensu stricto	Yes	US, Europe	*Ixodes scapularis, I pacificus, I ricinus*	Rodents, birds
B afzelii	Yes	Europe, Asia	*I ricinus, I persulcatus*	Rodents
B garinii	Yes	Europe, Asia	*I ricinus, I persulcatus*	Birds, rodents
B bavariensis	Yes	Europe, Asia	*I ricinus, I persulcatus*	Rodents
B americana	Cases reported	US	*I pacificus, I minor*	Birds
B andersonii	Cases reported	US	*I dentatus*	Cotton tail rabbit
B bissettii	Cases reported	US, Europe	*I scapularis, I pacificus, I ricinus, I minor*	Birds, rodents
B spielmanii	Cases reported	Europe	*I ricinus*	Rodents
B valaisiana	Cases reported	Europe, Asia	*I ricinus, I granulates*	Birds
B lusitaniae	Cases reported	Europe, North Africa	*I ricinus*	Rodents
B californiensis	No evidence to date	US	*I pacificus, I jellisonii, I spinipalpis*	Kangaroo rat, mule deer
B carolinensis	No evidence to date	US	*I minor*	Rodents
B kurtenbachii	No evidence to date	US, Europe	*I scapulatus*	Rodents
B finlandensis	No evidence to date	Finland	*I ricinus*	Unknown
B sinica	No evidence to date	China	*I ovatus*	Rodents
B yangtze	No evidence to date	China, Japan	*Haemaphysalis longicornis, I granulatus*	Rodents, shrews
B japonica	No evidence to date	Japan	*I ovatus*	Rodents
B tanukii	No evidence to date	Japan	*I tanuki*	Unknown
B turdi	No evidence to date	Japan	*I turdus*	Birds

Lyme disease is a zoonotic disease, meaning that the borreliae that cause disease are maintained by animal and tick populations, and humans are only incidentally infected when fed on by infected ticks (**Fig. 2**). The various genospecies of the spirochete complex vary in their abilities to infect and be maintained by different reservoir host species. Generalist members of the complex are able to successfully infect many phylogenetically distant hosts, whereas other more specialist members are only able

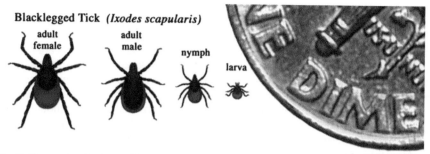

Fig. 2. The vector for Lyme disease in the eastern United States, *I scapularis*. The tick is also commonly referred to as the blacklegged (or deer) tick. All life stages of the tick are shown. (*From* Lyme Disease. Centers for Disease Control and Prevention. Available at: http://www. cdc.gov/lyme/index.html. Accessed September 9, 2015.)

to infect one or a few closely related host species. *B burgdorferi* in North America is a generalist that infects many vertebrate hosts, including mammals, birds, and reptiles.[32] Species in Europe, on the other hand, tend to be more specialized and infect certain groups of vertebrates. Generally, *B afzelii* infections are associated with rodents and some insectivore species, whereas *B garinii* tends to be maintained by birds and some rodents (see **Table 1**).[33,34]

THE VECTOR

Only ticks belonging to the hard tick genus *Ixodes* have been shown to be competent vectors for Lyme disease; thus, the geographic distribution of Lyme disease is limited to the natural territory of these ticks. There are 4 predominant species of *Ixodes* ticks that transmit disease to humans, including *Ixodes scapularis* in the eastern United States and Canada (**Fig. 3**), *Ixodes pacificus* in the western United States, *Ixodes ricinus* in Europe and Asia, and *Ixodes persulcatus* in Asia.[24,27] In the northeastern

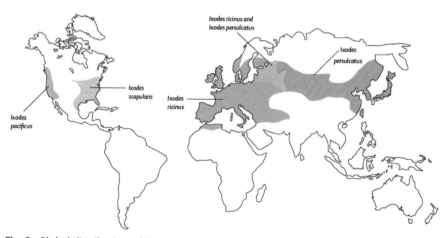

Fig. 3. Global distribution of the *Ixodes* species that are the primary vectors for Lyme borreliosis in humans. (*From* Stanek G, Wormser GP, Gray J, et al. Lyme borreliosis. Lancet 2012;379:461–73. *Adapted with permission from* the European Concerted Action on Lyme Borreliosis. Available at: http://www.eucalb.com/.)

United States, the vector was originally described as *Ixodes dammini*, a species distinct from *I scapularis*.[35] In the 1990s, studies demonstrated that the 2 forms were conspecific, resulting in *I dammini* being resynonymized with *I scapularis*.[36,37]

Ixodes ticks depend on vertebrate hosts to provide the blood meals that are necessary for them to reproduce and develop. Specifically, 3 blood meals, one for each life stage (larva, nymph, and adult), are required by the ticks to complete their life cycles. Development from larva to adult may take 1 to 4 years to complete, depending on climatic conditions and the availability of hosts, although it is generally thought that 2 years is the typical length of the *Ixodes* tick life cycle.[38] Between each developmental stage, following each blood meal, the ticks are independent of the host, and therefore, their survival and behavior are affected by environmental conditions. The ticks are particularly sensitive to drying conditions and require a relative humidity of at least 80%. They generally are restricted to areas of moderate to high rainfall with good soil drainage and vegetation.[38,39]

The ticks both acquire and transmit *B. burgdoferi* s.l by feeding on the vertebrate animals that act as the reservoir hosts for the pathogens. Experimental evidence has failed to demonstrate transovarial (eg, mother-to-egg) transmission[40,41]; larvae, therefore, are born uninfected. Once ticks become infected by feeding on an infected host, they retain the infection through the molting process that occurs between life stages, and consequently, they are capable of transmitting the spirochetes during the next blood meal (**Fig. 4**). This process is termed transstadial transmission.

The different stages of *Ixodes* ticks may feed on a wide variety of mammals, birds, and reptiles, but seem to have preferences for certain hosts, which vary geographically. For instance, although *I scapularis* ticks have been found on at least 30 types of wild animals and 71 species of birds,[42,43] most *I scapularis* larvae and nymphs in the northeastern United States feed on small mammals, including mice, chipmunks, and shrews.[44] By contrast, *I scapularis* larvae and nymphs in the southern United States are less inclined to feed on small rodents and are found to feed most frequently on lizards and skinks.[45,46] Larvae and nymphs of *I pacificus* in the western United States also feed predominately on a lizard, the western fence lizard (*Sceloporus occidentalis*).[47] Larger animals, including white-tailed deer (*Odocoileus virginianus*) in the eastern United States, mule deer (*Odocoileus heionus*) in the western United States, and various deer species (*Capreolus capreolus, Cervus elaphus*), and domestic sheep and cattle in Europe, play a central role as blood-meal sources for the adult stages of the ticks.[24,27]

Despite having preferences for certain hosts, the *Ixodes* species that are the primary vectors of Lyme disease worldwide (eg, *I scapularis, I ricinus,* and *I persulcatus*) are considered to be generalist feeders and that it is the generalist nature of the ticks that provide opportunities for transmission of borreliae to humans as well as between different types of host species, potentially linking the different ecological niches of the spirochetes.[48] The generalist nature of the ticks may also be an important mechanism for introducing *Borrelia* into new habitats and for causing illness in humans by atypical strains or genospecies; as such, *I scapularis* has been termed a bridging vector.[28,49] It is also possible that *Ixodes* species that are usually highly restrictive in their diets will occasionally feed on humans and infect humans with atypical strains or genospecies. For instance, *Borrelia andersonii*, a member of the Lyme borreliae group, is associated with the tick *Ixodes dentatus*, which feeds almost exclusively on birds and rabbits. It is known to rarely feed on humans, however,[50–52] and patients with a Lyme-like illness were recently identified with *B andersonii* infections in the United States.[29,53] Which tick species is more likely to transmit such atypical infections to humans is currently unknown.

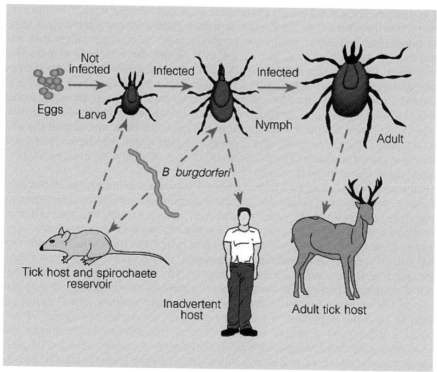

Fig. 4. Life cycle of the *Ixodes* tick vectors of Lyme borreliosis. Reservoir hosts, such as mice, transmit *B burgdorferi* to the larva or nymph stages of the tick when they take a blood meal. The spirochetes are then transmitted by infected nymphs or adult ticks to other reservoir hosts and to humans, which are inadvertent hosts. Deer are important hosts for adult ticks, but they are not effective reservoirs for *B burgdorferi*. (*From* Barbour AG, Zuckert WR. Genome sequencing: new tricks of tick-borne pathogen. Nature 1997;390:553; with permission.)

RESERVOIR HOSTS AND THE AMPLIFICATION OF *BORRELIA BURGDORFERI* S.L. IN NATURE

The capacity of an animal to serve as a reservoir host depends on the susceptibility of that host to the infectious agent as well as the ability of that host to disseminate the agent. The white-footed mouse (*Peromyscus leucopus*) is generally considered to be the most competent reservoir host for *B burgdorferi* in eastern North America. It is estimated that more than 90% of mice exposed to nymphs infected with *B burgdorferi* will become infected,[44,54] and between 75% and 95% of *I scapularis* larvae that feed on infected mice will become infected.[55] Once mice are infected, evidence suggests they remain infectious for life,[54,56] and because their survival does not seem to be negatively affected by infections,[57–59] infected mice are likely to transmit spirochetes to ticks many times during their lives. Therefore, given that mice are a preferred host for subadult ticks in eastern North America, in regions where they are abundant, mice are major contributors to the overall prevalence of *B burgdorferi*–infected ticks.[55,58] Indeed, where mice are the primary host available, nearly all infected nymphs will obtain their infections from mice (eg,[60]). Estimates from field studies conducted where mice exist with other potential reservoir hosts suggest only 25% to 35%

of infected nymphs acquire their spirochetes from white-footed mice.[58,59,61] In such mixed rodent communities, the Eastern chipmunk (Tamias striates) and shrews (Blarina brevicauda and Sorex spp) have been identified as reservoir hosts that also contribute significantly to the prevalence of B burgdorferi infections in ticks. For instance, in Dutchess County, New York, USA, where the ecology of Lyme disease has been studied extensively (eg,[55]), it was estimated that shrews had fed 55% of infected ticks; in contrast, 25% of infected ticks had been fed by white-footed mice.[61] However, the study conceded that nearly all infected nymphs (90%) took their larval blood meals from a limited subset of the potential hosts available at the site: white-footed mice, chipmunks, and shrews, suggesting that maintenance of Lyme disease in the northeastern United States will be most strongly dependent on the population dynamics of these few hosts.[61]

In the western and southern United States, the larvae and nymphs of Ixodes ticks display different feeding behaviors, and the B burgdorferi pathogen is maintained by other, less competent hosts, which may at least partially explain why risks of human infections in these regions are lower (eg, see **Fig. 1**). The western fence lizard, a refractory host, feeds most I pacificus larvae and nymphs in California, and although deer mice (Peromyscus maniculatus) are present, they do not appear to be important hosts for B burgdorferi; rather the western gray squirrel (Sciurus griseus) may be the most important reservoir host there.[62] Likewise, lizards feed most subadult ticks in the southern United States, and other rodent species, not P leucopus, seem to be more important in maintaining the B burgdorferi life cycle.[63] These life-cycle differences probably explain some of the differences in human risk observed across these regions, as a lower prevalence of infected ticks will be available to transmit infections to humans where subadult ticks prefer to feed on incompetent reservoir hosts.

Birds are recognized as important reservoir hosts for certain members of the B burgdorferi s.l complex. For instance, B garinii and B valaisiana in Europe and Asia are preferentially associated with bird reservoir hosts,[64,65] including several species of seabirds, which are thought to be involved in a global transmission cycle of B garinii.[66,67] In North America, 70 passerine species and one species of woodpecker have been reported as hosts for subadult stages of I scapularis, with ground-dwelling birds being particularly infested. Most passerine species examined also seem capable of becoming infected and transmitting B burgdorferi infections to I scapularis larvae.[43] It is still unclear how important birds are in maintaining local B burgdorferi transmission[68] or in contributing to the risk of transmission to humans, as prevalences of infections in birds and ticks recovered from birds are fairly low (<5%).[69,70] However, evidence does suggest that birds, especially migratory birds, may be significant drivers in the spread of I scapularis, and therefore, may be important contributors to the expansion of Lyme disease in North America.[71,72]

Deer and other large cervids, including domestic sheep in Europe, are generally considered to be critical hosts for the tick vectors of Lyme borreliosis.[73,74] All 3 life stages of I scapularis, for instance, are found in abundance on white-tailed deer in the eastern United States, with the adult stages of the tick exhibiting an especially strong dependence on these hosts. Recent work using host blood meal identification analyses confirmed that up to 40% of questing nymphs may have obtained their blood meals from deer.[75,76] Deer are, however, refractory to Borrelia infections, and therefore, are unlikely to transmit infections to ticks.[73,74,77] As such, deer play a significant role in the amplification of tick populations, but are not themselves involved in the infectious life cycle of Lyme disease. Deer have been blamed for the rapid intensification and spread of I scapularis and Lyme disease observed in recent decades in the eastern United States.[78] Their populations have grown in response to reforestation and protection from predation and hunting, and they are highly adaptable to suburban and even urban environments.

In addition to ticks acquiring infections directly from an infected blood meal, a process known as cofeeding transmission also has been described. In this mode of transmission, uninfected ticks acquire infections from infected ticks that are feeding in close proximity to them on the same host. The phenomenon has been demonstrated in transmission of *B burgdorferi* by *I scapularis*[79,80] and *I ricinus*,[81] *B afzelii* by *I ricinus*,[82] and *B garinii* by *I persulcatus*.[83] The significance of cofeeding transmission to the epidemiology of Lyme borreliosis is poorly understood; however, it seems to be more efficient in the European system of *B afzelii* and *I ricinus* than the North American system of *B burgdorferi* and *I scapularis*.[84] The importance is related to the potential for nymph-to-larva cofeeding events, which depends on the synchrony of larval and nymphal host searching and questing activity. In Europe, the 2 stages of immature ticks are active during the same times of year from spring to autumn, whereas in North America, the peak activity of the stages may occur during different times of year.[48,85] Because deer and other large cervids may carry all stages of ticks simultaneously, these hosts may play an important role in providing a platform for cofeeding transmission to occur even though they are not infected themselves.[84]

SEASONALITY OF TICK ACTIVITY AND HUMAN INFECTIONS

Because the larvae of *Ixodes* ticks are not yet infected with *B burgdorferi*, transmission of infections to humans is associated primarily with the nymph or adult stages of the ticks. Defining the activity patterns of the different tick life stages relative to when humans acquire infections, therefore, is important for identifying the stage most likely to transmit infections to humans and to guide efforts to control the disease in humans. Although many studies have been done since the discovery of Lyme disease to reveal the natural history of the tick life cycle, details of the patterns of seasonal activity remain unknown or incomplete. Confusion stems from variation in activity patterns that have been observed for the different tick life stages in relation to climate and geography. In Europe, early studies of *I ricinus* revealed bimodal seasonal patterns for the 3 life stages (larva, nymph, adult), whereas in North America, the activity patterns of *I scapularis* are predominately unimodal (**Fig. 5**). In general, on both continents, adults become active early in the spring when temperatures exceed 44°F (7°C).[38] Female ticks that overwinter in a fed state may commence to lay eggs at this time; otherwise, adults will begin host seeking, also known as questing, for a blood meal, feed, reproduce, and then lay eggs. Thus, there tends to be one peak in adult activity in the spring. Nymphs will also become active and begin questing in the spring with their peaks in the spring or early summer. Some of these nymphs will successfully feed and molt into adults that same year, and therefore, there typically is a second peak of adult activity in the fall of each year. In Europe, second peaks of *I ricinus* nymphs may be observed in the fall, although second peaks are not observed for *I scapularis* in North America. Timing of larval activity and peak abundances also vary. As for nymphs of *I ricinus* in Europe, larvae may have one period of activity in late spring to early summer, followed by a second period in the fall. For *I scapularis* in the northeastern United States, peak larval activity occurs in late summer to early fall. However, in the Midwestern United States, evidence suggests emergence and peak activity of *I scapularis* larvae occur in the spring and early summer (see **Fig. 5**).[85,86]

It is understood that the seasonal activity of the various life stages relative to each other is critical for the ecology and epidemiology of Lyme disease. The

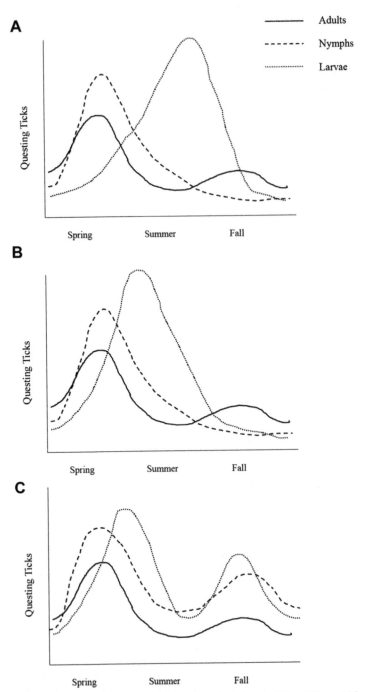

Fig. 5. Generalized seasonal activity of the relative abundance of the different life stages of *Ixodes* ticks. Variation in activity is observed geographically. In the United States, activity patterns of larvae and nymphs tend to be unimodal, although 2 peaks, one in spring and one in fall, are observed for adult ticks (*A* and *B*). In the northeastern United States, peak activities tend to be fairly discrete, with peak nymph activity in late spring or early summer and peak larvae activity in late summer or early fall (*A*), whereas activity of nymphs and larvae seems to be more overlapping in the Midwestern United States (*B*). Bimodal activity patterns are observed for all life stages of *I ricinus* in Europe (*C*).

year-to-year perpetuation of *B burgdorferi* depends on larvae feeding after infected nymphs have transmitted the pathogens to reservoir hosts. This pattern of activity results in larvae effectively acquiring the spirochete such that a population of infected nymphs will be available to transmit infections to a new cohort of reservoir hosts the following year.[48] How much overlap there is in the activity of the nymphs and larvae will also be important for determining the relevance of cofeeding to disease transmission.[84]

Because the spring and early summer peak activity periods of nymphs coincide with when humans are most likely to become infected (see **Fig. 5**; **Fig. 6**), it is thought that this tick stage is the most important stage for transmission of Lyme disease to humans. The small size of the nymph and its ability to go undetected while feeding on humans also likely contributes to the significance of nymphs as vectors of Lyme disease in humans. As a consequence, the density of nymphs, nymphal infection prevalence, and the density of infected nymphs are often used as indicators of human infection risk in an area.[55,87,88] However, it should be noted that infections can also be acquired by adult ticks, and it may be the adult stage that is more associated with human infections acquired in the fall (see **Fig. 6**).

GENETIC FACTORS

Genetic factors play a role in the pathogenicity of the organism. *B afzelii* causes primary skin manifestations, including erythema migrans (EM) and acrodermatitis chronica atrophicans, *B garnii* infections are often associated with neurologic manifestations, and joint pain and swelling are particularly associated with *B burgdorferi* infections.[23,24,89,90] Two genetic markers of *B burgdorferi*, ribosome spacer type (RST) and outer surface protein C (ospC) have been used for genotyping. RST typing using restriction fragment length polymorphism divides *B burgdorferi* into 3 types. RST 1 is more likely to disseminate, cause severe disease, cause increased inflammation, and lead to refractory arthritis. RST 2 causes intermediate symptoms, and RST 3 produces the least severe symptoms.[90–96] Typing of ospC region produces 21 unique

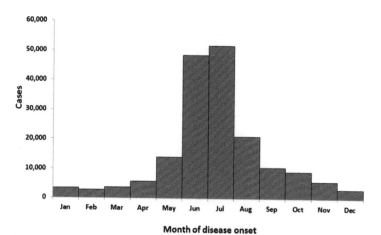

Fig. 6. Confirmed Lyme disease cases by month of disease onset in the United States, 2001 to 2010. (*From* Lyme Disease. Centers for Disease Control and Prevention. Available at: http://www.cdc.gov/lyme/stats/chartstables/casesbymonth.html. Accessed September 9, 2015.)

types, 16 of which have been identified in the northeastern United States. It is likely that all types have the ability to disseminate; however, types A, B, I, and H have the greatest tendency to disseminate. Type K, followed by type A, is the most common type in the United States, resulting in the most disseminated infections.[23,91–95,97–99] There is strong correlation between RST and ospC typing (**Table 2**).[91,94,95] Recent studies using multilocus sequence typing of B burgdorferi have shown similar patterns of virulence and strong, although not complete, correlation to ospC typing.[100] Phylogenetic studies show high heterogeneity of B burgdorferi in the United States and Canada,[20,97] and different ospC types tend to be associated with particular reservoir hosts[101]; therefore, the ecology of Lyme disease, and the variants that are naturally circulating in a collection of available hosts, will influence the severity of illnesses observed regionally.[22,100]

LYME DISEASE IN THE SOUTHERN UNITED STATES

Lyme disease transmission dynamics and the risks to humans in southern states are still poorly understood. Cases of Lyme disease are reported to the CDC, and the numbers of cases, as elsewhere in the United States, are growing. Southern patients do present with EM-like rashes and other symptoms similar to those observed in Lyme disease patients; however, the causative agent or agents of the illness in these patients have not been clearly identified. Attempts to culture Borrelia organisms from skin biopsies obtained from affected patients have failed, and serologic tests rarely support exposure to B burgdorferi.[102–104] The EM-like rashes and illness in these patients also have frequently been associated with bites from the lone star tick, Amblyomma americanum, which is the predominant human-biting tick in the southern United States,[63,105] rather than bites of I scapularis.[53,106] Despite these associations, efforts to isolate B burgdorferi from A americanum using culture and molecular assays have failed to provide evidence that these ticks consistently carry

Table 2 Correlation of RST and *ospC* genotypes of Lyme *Borrelia*	
RST Genotype	***ospC* Genotype**
1	A[a,b] B[a]
2	F H[a] K[a,b] N
3	C D E G I[a] J M O T U

[a] Most virulent genotypes.
[b] Most common genotypes.

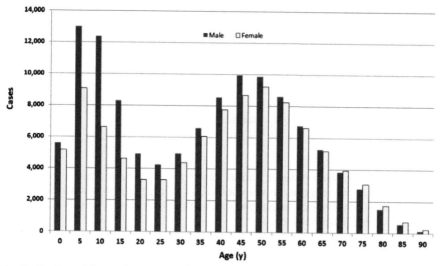

Fig. 7. Confirmed Lyme disease cases by age and sex in the United States, 2001 to 2010. (*From* Lyme Disease. Centers for Disease Control and Prevention. Available at: http://www. cdc.gov/lyme/stats/chartstables/incidencebyagesex.html.)

infections,[107] and laboratory trials have failed to demonstrate the tick's ability to transmit infections.[108,109] A tick relapsing fever group *Borrelia* species, identified as *Borrelia lonestari*, was investigated as the possible cause of Lyme-like illness in the southern United States, because it has frequently been found in *A americanum* ticks.[110] However, only one reported case of an early Lyme-like illness has been associated with *B lonestari* infection. In this patient, *B lonestari* DNA was isolated from the skin of an EM-like rash and an attached *A americanum* tick associated with the case.[111] *B burgdorferi* has been isolated from *Ixodes affinis* and rodent hosts in the coastal areas of the southern United States, but it is not clear how often humans may be bitten by these ticks and infected with *B burgdorferi*.[112] Investigations by Clark and colleagues[29,53] suggest other *B burgdorferi* s.l. species may cause disease in people in southern states, although their findings will have to be confirmed by others (see Ref.[107]).

RISK FACTORS FOR LYME DISEASE

Lyme disease has a bimodal age distribution with peaks at ages 5 to 15 and 45 to 59 (**Fig. 7**).[14,113–118] The number of reported cases in the United States is highest among boys aged 5 to 9.[14] A shift in more infections in men has been observed in recent years.[8]

Numerous studies have examined factors that place individuals at increased risk for Lyme disease. Living and working in endemic areas or in close association with suitable tick habitats, especially forested or shrub habitats, are important factors for adults and children.[119–121] Number of hours spent outdoors has a strong correlation with Lyme disease risk.[118,122,123] Protective clothing can protect from infection. Repellents, checking the body for ticks after outdoor activities, and showering within 2 hours of outdoor activities have consistently shown to be of benefit.[24,124–127]

SELF-ASSESSMENT

1. A bite by which tick life stage is thought to be most frequently associated with transmission of Lyme borreliosis to humans?
   A. Larva
   B. Nymph
   C. Adult female
   D. Adult male
2. Globally, the incidence of Lyme disease is:
   A. Stable
   B. Decreasing
   C. Increasing
   D. Increasing in North America and decreasing in Europe and Asia
3. A patient presents to a clinic in Vermont, USA with erythema migrans in June, with no history of travel. Which of the following natural tick–reservoir host life cycles did the patient most likely intercept?
   A. *Ixodes scapularis*—lizard
   B. *Ixodes scapularis*—white-footed mouse
   C. *Ixodes pacificus*—deer mouse
   D. *Ixodes ricinus*—domestic sheep
4. Cases of Lyme disease in Europe are caused by which species?
   A. *B burgdorferi*
   B. *B afzelii*
   C. *B garinii*
   D. *B burgdorferi, B afzelii,* and *B garinii*
5. All of the following statements with regards to the epidemiology of Lyme disease are true, EXCEPT:
   A. Lyme disease occurs primarily in the late fall.
   B. Lyme disease has a bimodal age distribution.
   C. Most Lyme disease cases occur in boys aged 5 to 14.
   D. There are 2 main areas of high incidence in humans in the United States located in the northeast and upper Midwest.

Answers
   Answer 1: B; Header cross-references: Seasonality of Tick Activity and Human Infections.
   Answer 2: C; Header cross-reference: Introduction.
   Answer 3: B; Header cross-references: Reservoir Hosts and the Amplification of *Borrelia burgdorferi* s.l. in Nature.
   Answer 4: D; Header cross-references: The Etiologic Agent and **Table 1**.
   Answer 5: A; Header cross-references: Risk Factors for Lyme Disease, **Figs. 1, 6,** and **7**.

REFERENCES

1. Steere AC, Malawista SE, Snydman DR, et al. Lyme arthritis: an epidemic of oligoarticular arthritis in children and adults in three connecticut communities. Arthritis Rheum 1977;20:7–17.
2. Steere AC. Lyme disease. N Engl J Med 1989;321:586–96.
3. Lindgren E, Jaenson TGT. Lyme borreliosis in Europe: influences of climate and climate change, epidemiology, ecology and adaptation measures. Geneva (Switzerland): World Health Organization; 2006.

4. Centers for Disease Control and Prevention. Summary of notifiable diseases–United States, 2012. MMWR Morb Mortal Wkly Rep 2014;61:124.
5. Mead PS. Epidemiology of Lyme disease. Infect Dis Clin North Am 2015;29:187–210.
6. Smith R, Takkinen J. Lyme borreliosis: Europe-wide coordinated surveillance and action needed? Euro Surveill 2006;11:E060622.1.
7. Kugeler KJ, Farley GM, Forrester DJ, et al. Geographic distribution and expansion of human Lyme disease, United States. Emerg Infect Dis 2015;21:1455–7.
8. Bacon RM, Kugeler KJ, Mead PS. Surveillance for Lyme disease–United States, 1992-2006. MMWR Surveill Summ 2008;57:1–9.
9. Rizzoli A, Hauffe H, Carpi G, et al. Lyme borreliosis in Europe. Euro Surveill 2011;16(27):19906.
10. Dehnert M, Fingerle V, Klier C, et al. Seropositivity of Lyme borreliosis and associated risk factors: a population-based study in children and adolescents in Germany (KiGGS). PLoS One 2012;7:e41321.
11. Skogman BH, Ekerfelt C, Ludvigsson J, et al. Seroprevalence of *Borrelia* IgG antibodies among young Swedish children in relation to reported tick bites, symptoms and previous treatment for Lyme borreliosis: a population-based survey. Arch Dis Child 2010;95:1013–6.
12. Chmielewska-Badora J, Moniuszko A, Zukiewicz-Sobczak W, et al. Serological survey in persons occupationally exposed to tick-borne pathogens in cases of co-infections with *Borrelia burgdorferi, Anaplasma phagocytophilum, Bartonella* spp. and *Babesia microti*. Ann Agric Environ Med 2012;19:271–4.
13. Dessau RB, Bangsborg JM, Ejlertsen T, et al. Utilization of serology for the diagnosis of suspected Lyme borreliosis in Denmark: survey of patients seen in general practice. BMC Infect Dis 2010;10:317.
14. Centers for Disease Control and Prevention. Lyme Disease. Available at: http://www.cdc.gov/lyme/. Accessed August 4, 2015.
15. Ogden NH, Koffi JK, Pelcat Y, et al. Environmental risk from Lyme disease in central and eastern Canada: a summary of recent surveillance information. Can Commun Dis Rep 2014;40:74–82. Available at: http://www.phac-aspc.gc.ca/publicat/ccdr-rmtc/14vol40/dr-rm40-05/index-eng.php. Accessed August 4, 2015.
16. Wilking H, Stark K. Trends in surveillance data of human Lyme borreliosis from six federal states in eastern Germany, 2009-2012. Ticks Tick Borne Dis 2014;5:219–24.
17. Hofhuis A, van der Giessen JW, Borgsteede FH, et al. Lyme borreliosis in the Netherlands: strong increase in GP consultations and hospital admissions in past 10 years. Euro Surveill 2006;11:E060622.2.
18. Gray JS, Dautel H, Estrada-Pena A, et al. Effects of climate change on ticks and tick-borne diseases in Europe. Interdiscip Perspect Infect Dis 2009;2009:593232.
19. Jore S, Vanwambeke SO, Viljugrein H, et al. Climate and environmental change drives *Ixodes ricinus* geographical expansion at the northern range margin. Parasit Vectors 2014;7:11.
20. Mechai S, Margos G, Feil EJ, et al. Complex population structure of *Borrelia burgdorferi* in southeastern and south central Canada as revealed by phylogeographic analysis. Appl Environ Microbiol 2015;81:1309–18.
21. Qiu WG, Bruno JF, McCaig WD, et al. Wide distribution of a high-virulence *Borrelia burgdorferi* clone in Europe and North America. Emerg Infect Dis 2008;14:1097–104.

22. Brisson D, Vandermause MF, Meece JK, et al. Evolution of northeastern and midwestern *Borrelia burgdorferi*, United States. Emerg Infect Dis 2010;16:911–7.

23. Baranton G, De Martino SJ. *Borrelia burgdorferi* sensu lato diversity and its influence on pathogenicity in humans. Curr Probl Dermatol 2009;37:1–17.

24. Stanek G, Wormser GP, Gray J, et al. Lyme borreliosis. Lancet 2012;379:461–73.

25. Rudenko N, Golovchenko M, Grubhoffer L, et al. Updates on *Borrelia burgdorferi* sensu lato complex with respect to public health. Ticks Tick Borne Dis 2011; 2:123–8.

26. Ruzic-Sabljic E, Maraspin V, Lotric-Furlan S, et al. Characterization of *Borrelia burgdorferi* sensu lato strains isolated from human material in Slovenia. Wien Klin Wochenschr 2002;114:544–50.

27. Piesman J, Gern L. Lyme borreliosis in Europe and North America. Parasitology 2004;129(Suppl):S191–220.

28. Girard YA, Fedorova N, Lane RS. Genetic diversity of *Borrelia burgdorferi* and detection of *B. bissettii*-like DNA in serum of north-coastal California residents. J Clin Microbiol 2011;49:945–54.

29. Clark KL, Leydet BF, Threlkeld C. Geographical and genospecies distribution of *Borrelia burgdorferi* sensu lato DNA detected in humans in the USA. J Med Microbiol 2014;63:674–84.

30. Casjens SR, Fraser-Liggett CM, Mongodin EF, et al. Whole genome sequence of an unusual *Borrelia burgdorferi* sensu lato isolate. J Bacteriol 2011;193: 1489–90.

31. Stanek G, Reiter M. The expanding Lyme Borrelia complex–clinical significance of genomic species? Clin Microbiol Infect 2011;17:487–93.

32. Hanincova K, Kurtenbach K, Diuk-Wasser M, et al. Epidemic spread of Lyme borreliosis, northeastern United States. Emerg Infect Dis 2006;12:604–11.

33. Hanincova K, Schafer SM, Etti S, et al. Association of *Borrelia afzelii* with rodents in Europe. Parasitology 2003;126:11–20.

34. Hanincova K, Taragelova V, Koci J, et al. Association of *Borrelia garinii* and *B. valaisiana* with songbirds in Slovakia. Appl Environ Microbiol 2003;69: 2825–30.

35. Spielman A, Clifford CM, Piesman J, et al. Human babesiosis on Nantucket Island, USA: description of the vector, *Ixodes (Ixodes) dammini*, n. sp. (Acarina: Ixodidae). J Med Entomol 1979;15:218–34.

36. Oliver JH Jr, Owsley MR, Hutcheson HJ, et al. Conspecificity of the ticks *Ixodes scapularis* and *I. dammini* (Acari: Ixodidae). J Med Entomol 1993;30:54–63.

37. Wesson DM, McLain DK, Oliver JH, et al. Investigation of the validity of species status of *Ixodes dammini* (Acari: Ixodidae) using rDNA. Proc Natl Acad Sci U S A 1993;90:10221–5.

38. Sonenshine DE. Ecology of non-nidicolous ticks. In: Sonenshine DE, editor. Biology of ticks. New York: Oxford University Press; 1993. p. 3–65.

39. Cortinas MR, Guerra MA, Jones CJ, et al. Detection, characterization, and prediction of tick-borne disease foci. Int J Med Microbiol 2002;291(Suppl 33): 11–20.

40. Richter D, Debski A, Hubalek Z, et al. Absence of Lyme disease spirochetes in larval *Ixodes ricinus* ticks. Vector Borne Zoonotic Dis 2012;12:21–7.

41. Rollend L, Fish D, Childs JE. Transovarial transmission of *Borrelia* spirochetes by *Ixodes scapularis*: a summary of the literature and recent observations. Ticks Tick Borne Dis 2013;4:46–51.

42. Anderson JF. Mammalian and avian reservoirs for *Borrelia burgdorferi*. Ann N Y Acad Sci 1988;539:180–91.

43. Brinkerhoff RJ, Folsom-O'Keefe CM, Tsao K, et al. Do birds affect Lyme disease risk? Range expansion of the vector-borne pathogen *Borrelia burgdorferi*. Front Ecol Environ 2011;9:103–10.
44. LoGiudice K, Ostfeld RS, Schmidt KA, et al. The ecology of infectious disease: effects of host diversity and community composition on Lyme disease risk. Proc Natl Acad Sci U S A 2003;100:567–71.
45. Apperson CS, Levine JF, Evans TL, et al. Relative utilization of reptiles and rodents as hosts by immature *Ixodes scapularis* (Acari: Ixodidae) in the coastal plain of North Carolina, USA. Exp Appl Acarol 1993;17:719–31.
46. Kollars TM Jr, Oliver JH Jr, Kollars PG, et al. Seasonal activity and host associations of *Ixodes scapularis* (Acari: Ixodidae) in southeastern Missouri. J Med Entomol 1999;36:720–6.
47. Eisen L, Eisen RJ, Lane RS. The roles of birds, lizards, and rodents as hosts for the western black-legged tick Ixodes pacificus. J Vector Ecol 2004;29: 295–308.
48. Kurtenbach K, Hanincova K, Tsao JI, et al. Fundamental processes in the evolutionary ecology of Lyme borreliosis. Nat Rev Microbiol 2006;4:660–9.
49. Hamer SA, Tsao JI, Walker ED, et al. Invasion of the Lyme disease vector *Ixodes scapularis*: implications for *Borrelia burgdorferi* endemicity. Ecohealth 2010;7: 47–63.
50. Walker ED, Stobierski MG, Poplar ML, et al. Geographic distribution of ticks (Acari: Ixodidae) in Michigan, with emphasis on *Ixodes scapularis* and *Borrelia burgdorferi*. J Med Entomol 1998;35:872–82.
51. Harrison BA, Engber BR, Apperson CS. Ticks (Acari: Ixodida) uncommonly found biting humans in North Carolina. J Vector Ecol 1997;22:6–12.
52. Anderson JF, Flavell RA, Magnarelli LA, et al. Novel *Borrelia burgdorferi* isolates from *Ixodes scapularis* and *Ixodes dentatus* ticks feeding on humans. J Clin Microbiol 1996;34:524–9.
53. Clark KL, Leydet B, Hartman S. Lyme borreliosis in human patients in Florida and Georgia, USA. Int J Med Sci 2013;10:915–31.
54. Donahue JG, Piesman J, Spielman A. Reservoir competence of white-footed mice for Lyme disease spirochetes. Am J Trop Med Hyg 1987;36:92–6.
55. Ostfeld RS. Lyme disease: the ecology of a complex system. New York: Oxford University Press, Inc; 2011.
56. Shih CM, Liu LP, Spielman A. Differential spirochetal infectivities to vector ticks of mice chronically infected by the agent of Lyme disease. J Clin Microbiol 1995; 33:3164–8.
57. Hofmeister EK, Ellis BA, Glass GE, et al. Longitudinal study of infection with *Borrelia burgdorferi* in a population of Peromyscus leucopus at a Lyme disease-enzootic site in Maryland. Am J Trop Med Hyg 1999;60:598–609.
58. Tsao JI, Wootton JT, Bunikis J, et al. An ecological approach to preventing human infection: vaccinating wild mouse reservoirs intervenes in the Lyme disease cycle. Proc Natl Acad Sci U S A 2004;101:18159–64.
59. Voordouw MJ, Lachish S, Dolan MC. The Lyme disease pathogen has no effect on the survival of its rodent reservoir host. PLoS One 2015;10: e0118265.
60. Mather TN, Wilson ML, Moore SI, et al. Comparing the relative potential of rodents as reservoirs of the Lyme disease spirochete (*Borrelia burgdorferi*). Am J Epidemiol 1989;130:143–50.
61. Brisson D, Dykhuizen DE, Ostfeld RS. Conspicuous impacts of inconspicuous hosts on the Lyme disease epidemic. Proc Biol Sci 2008;275:227–35.

62. Eisen L, Eisen RJ, Mun J, et al. Transmission cycles of *Borrelia burgdorferi* and *B. bissettii* in relation to habitat type in northwestern California. J Vector Ecol 2009;34:81–91.

63. Stromdahl EY, Hickling GJ. Beyond Lyme: aetiology of tick-borne human diseases with emphasis on the south-eastern United States. Zoonoses Public Health 2012;59(Suppl 2):48–64.

64. Kurtenbach K, Peacey M, Rijpkema SG, et al. Differential transmission of the genospecies of *Borrelia burgdorferi* sensu lato by game birds and small rodents in England. Appl Environ Microbiol 1998;64:1169–74.

65. Kurtenbach K, De Michelis S, Etti S, et al. Host association of *Borrelia burgdorferi* sensu lato–the key role of host complement. Trends Microbiol 2002;10: 74–9.

66. Olsen B, Duffy DC, Jaenson TG, et al. Transhemispheric exchange of Lyme disease spirochetes by seabirds. J Clin Microbiol 1995;33:3270–4.

67. Comstedt P, Asokliene L, Eliasson I, et al. Complex population structure of Lyme borreliosis group spirochete *Borrelia garinii* in subarctic Eurasia. PLoS One 2009;4:e5841.

68. Giardina AR, Schmidt KA, Schauber EM, et al. Modeling the role of songbirds and rodents in the ecology of Lyme disease. Can J Zool 2000;78:2184–97.

69. Ogden NH, Lindsay LR, Hanincova K, et al. Role of migratory birds in introduction and range expansion of Ixodes scapularis ticks and of *Borrelia burgdorferi* and *Anaplasma phagocytophilum* in Canada. Appl Environ Microbiol 2008;74: 1780–90.

70. Brinkerhoff RJ, Folsom-O'Keefe CM, Streby HM, et al. Regional variation in immature *Ixodes scapularis* parasitism on North American songbirds: implications for transmission of the Lyme pathogen, *Borrelia burgdorferi*. J Med Entomol 2011;48:422–8.

71. Ogden NH, Trudel L, Artsob H, et al. *Ixodes scapularis* ticks collected by passive surveillance in Canada: analysis of geographic distribution and infection with Lyme borreliosis agent *Borrelia burgdorferi*. J Med Entomol 2006;43:600–9.

72. Ogden NH, Barker IK, Francis CA, et al. How far north are migrant birds transporting the tick *Ixodes scapularis* in Canada? Insights from stable hydrogen isotope analyses of feathers. Ticks Tick Borne Dis 2015, in press.

73. Jaenson TG, Talleklint L. Incompetence of roe deer as reservoirs of the Lyme borreliosis spirochete. J Med Entomol 1992;29:813–7.

74. Matuschka FR, Heiler M, Eiffert H, et al. Diversionary role of hoofed game in the transmission of Lyme disease spirochetes. Am J Trop Med Hyg 1993;48:693–9.

75. Moran Cadenas F, Rais O, Humair PF, et al. Identification of host bloodmeal source and *Borrelia burgdorferi* sensu lato in field-collected *Ixodes ricinus* ticks in Chaumont (Switzerland). J Med Entomol 2007;44:1109–17.

76. Scott MC, Harmon JR, Tsao JI, et al. Reverse line blot probe design and polymerase chain reaction optimization for bloodmeal analysis of ticks from the eastern United States. J Med Entomol 2012;49:697–709.

77. Telford SR 3rd, Mather TN, Moore SI, et al. Incompetence of deer as reservoirs of the Lyme disease spirochete. Am J Trop Med Hyg 1988;39:105–9.

78. Spielman A, Wilson ML, Levine JF, et al. Ecology of *Ixodes dammini*-borne human babesiosis and Lyme disease. Annu Rev Entomol 1985;30:439–60.

79. Patrican LA. Acquisition of Lyme disease spirochetes by cofeeding Ixodes scapularis ticks. Am J Trop Med Hyg 1997;57:589–93.

80. Piesman J, Happ CM. The efficacy of co-feeding as a means of maintaining *Borrelia burgdorferi*: a North American model system. J Vector Ecol 2001;26:216–20.

81. Gern L, Rais O. Efficient transmission of *Borrelia burgdorferi* between cofeeding *Ixodes ricinus* ticks (Acari: Ixodidae). J Med Entomol 1996;33:189–92.
82. Richter D, Allgower R, Matuschka FR. Co-feeding transmission and its contribution to the perpetuation of the Lyme disease spirochete *Borrelia afzelii*. Emerg Infect Dis 2002;8:1421–5.
83. Sato Y, Nakao M. Transmission of the Lyme disease spirochete, *Borrelia garinii*, between infected and uninfected immature *Ixodes persulcatus* during cofeeding on mice. J Parasitol 1997;83:547–50.
84. Voordouw MJ. Co-feeding transmission in Lyme disease pathogens. Parasitology 2015;142:290–302.
85. Gatewood AG, Liebman KA, Vourc'h G, et al. Climate and tick seasonality are predictors of *Borrelia burgdorferi* genotype distribution. Appl Environ Microbiol 2009;75:2476–83.
86. Johnson RC, Kodner C, Jarnefeld J, et al. Agents of human anaplasmosis and Lyme disease at Camp Ripley, Minnesota. Vector Borne Zoonotic Dis 2011; 11(12):1529–34.
87. Mather TN, Nicholson MC, Donnelly EF, et al. Entomologic index for human risk of Lyme disease. Am J Epidemiol 1996;144:1066–9.
88. Stafford KC 3rd, Cartter ML, Magnarelli LA, et al. Temporal correlations between tick abundance and prevalence of ticks infected with *Borrelia burgdorferi* and increasing incidence of Lyme disease. J Clin Microbiol 1998;36:1240–4.
89. Dubrey SW, Bhatia A, Woodham S, et al. Lyme disease in the United Kingdom. Postgrad Med J 2014;90:33–42.
90. Wang G, van Dam AP, Schwartz I, et al. Molecular typing of *Borrelia burgdorferi* sensu lato: taxonomic, epidemiological, and clinical implications. Clin Microbiol Rev 1999;12:633–53.
91. Jones KL, Glickstein LJ, Damle N, et al. *Borrelia burgdorferi* genetic markers and disseminated disease in patients with early Lyme disease. J Clin Microbiol 2006;44:4407–13.
92. Jones KL, McHugh GA, Glickstein LJ, et al. Analysis of *Borrelia burgdorferi* genotypes in patients with Lyme arthritis: high frequency of ribosomal RNA intergenic spacer type 1 strains in antibiotic-refractory arthritis. Arthritis Rheum 2009;60:2174–82.
93. Strle K, Jones KL, Drouin EE, et al. *Borrelia burgdorferi* RST1 (OspC type A) genotype is associated with greater inflammation and more severe Lyme disease. Am J Pathol 2011;178:2726–39.
94. Wang G, Ojaimi C, Wu H, et al. Disease severity in a murine model of Lyme borreliosis is associated with the genotype of the infecting *Borrelia burgdorferi* sensu stricto strain. J Infect Dis 2002;186:782–91.
95. Wormser GP, Brisson D, Liveris D, et al. *Borrelia burgdorferi* genotype predicts the capacity for hematogenous dissemination during early Lyme disease. J Infect Dis 2008;198:1358–64.
96. Wormser GP, Liveris D, Nowakowski J, et al. Association of specific subtypes of *Borrelia burgdorferi* with hematogenous dissemination in early Lyme disease. J Infect Dis 1999;180:720–5.
97. Brisson D, Baxamusa N, Schwartz I, et al. Biodiversity of *Borrelia burgdorferi* strains in tissues of Lyme disease patients. PLoS One 2011;6:e22926.
98. Dykhuizen DE, Brisson D, Sandigursky S, et al. The propensity of different *Borrelia burgdorferi* sensu stricto genotypes to cause disseminated infections in humans. Am J Trop Med Hyg 2008;78:806–10.

99. Tijsse-Klasen E, Pandak N, Hengeveld P, et al. Ability to cause erythema migrans differs between *Borrelia burgdorferi* sensu lato isolates. Parasit Vectors 2013;6:23.
100. Hanincova K, Mukherjee P, Ogden NH, et al. Multilocus sequence typing of *Borrelia burgdorferi* suggests existence of lineages with differential pathogenic properties in humans. PLoS One 2013;8:e73066.
101. Brisson D, Dykhuizen DE. ospC diversity in *Borrelia burgdorferi*: different hosts are different niches. Genetics 2004;168:713–22.
102. Campbell GL, Paul WS, Schriefer ME, et al. Epidemiologic and diagnostic studies of patients with suspected early Lyme disease, Missouri, 1990-1993. J Infect Dis 1995;172:470–80.
103. Wormser GP, Masters E, Nowakowski J, et al. Prospective clinical evaluation of patients from Missouri and New York with erythema migrans-like skin lesions. Clin Infect Dis 2005;41:958–65.
104. Philipp MT, Masters E, Wormser GP, et al. Serologic evaluation of patients from Missouri with erythema migrans-like skin lesions with the C6 Lyme test. Clin Vaccin Immunol 2006;13:1170–1.
105. Merten HA, Durden LA. A state-by-state survey of ticks recorded from humans in the United States. J Vector Ecol 2000;25:102–13.
106. Masters EJ, Grigery CN, Masters RW. STARI, or Masters disease: Lone Star tick-vectored Lyme-like illness. Infect Dis Clin North Am 2008;22:361–76, viii.
107. Stromdahl EY, Nadolny RM, Gibbons JA, et al. *Borrelia burgdorferi* not confirmed in human-biting *Amblyomma americanum* ticks from the southeastern United States. J Clin Microbiol 2015;53:1697–704.
108. Piesman J, Sinsky RJ. Ability to *Ixodes scapularis*, *Dermacentor variabilis*, and *Amblyomma americanum* (Acari: Ixodidae) to acquire, maintain, and transmit Lyme disease spirochetes (*Borrelia burgdorferi*). J Med Entomol 1988;25:336–9.
109. Piesman J, Happ CM. Ability of the Lyme disease spirochete *Borrelia burgdorferi* to infect rodents and three species of human-biting ticks (blacklegged tick, American dog tick, lone star tick) (Acari: Ixodidae). J Med Entomol 1997;34:451–6.
110. Barbour AG, Maupin GO, Teltow GJ, et al. Identification of an uncultivable *Borrelia* species in the hard tick *Amblyomma americanum*: possible agent of a Lyme disease-like illness. J Infect Dis 1996;173:403–9.
111. James AM, Liveris D, Wormser GP, et al. *Borrelia lonestari* infection after a bite by an *Amblyomma americanum* tick. J Infect Dis 2001;183:1810–4.
112. Rudenko N, Golovchenko M, Honig V, et al. Detection of *Borrelia burgdorferi* sensu stricto ospC alleles associated with human Lyme borreliosis worldwide in non-human-biting tick *Ixodes affinis* and rodent hosts in southeastern United States. Appl Environ Microbiol 2013;79:1444–53.
113. Bennet L, Stjernberg L, Berglund J. Effect of gender on clinical and epidemiologic features of Lyme borreliosis. Vector Borne Zoonotic Dis 2007;7:34–41.
114. Fulop B, Poggensee G. Epidemiological situation of Lyme borreliosis in Germany: surveillance data from six Eastern German States, 2002 to 2006. Parasitol Res 2008;103(Suppl 1):S117–20.
115. Lohr B, Muller I, Mai M, et al. Epidemiology and cost of hospital care for Lyme borreliosis in Germany: lessons from a health care utilization database analysis. Ticks Tick Borne Dis 2015;6:56–62.
116. Centers for Disease Control and Prevention. Surveillance for Lyme disease-United States. MMWR Morb Mortal Wkly Rep 2010;57:1–9.

117. Shapiro ED. *Borrelia burgdorferi* (Lyme disease). Pediatr Rev 2014;35:500–9.
118. Smith G, Wileyto EP, Hopkins RB, et al. Risk factors for Lyme disease in Chester County, Pennsylvania. Public Health Rep 2001;116(Suppl 1):146–56.
119. Killilea ME, Swei A, Lane RS, et al. Spatial dynamics of Lyme disease: a review. Ecohealth 2008;5:167–95.
120. Klein JD, Eppes SC, Hunt P. Environmental and life-style risk factors for Lyme disease in children. Clin Pediatr (Phila) 1996;35:359–63.
121. Connally NP, Ginsberg HS, Mather TN. Assessing peridomestic entomological factors as predictors for Lyme disease. J Vector Ecol 2006;31:364–70.
122. Cook MJ. Lyme borreliosis: a review of data on transmission time after tick attachment. Int J Gen Med 2015;8:1–8.
123. Finch C, Al-Damluji MS, Krause PJ, et al. Integrated assessment of behavioral and environmental risk factors for Lyme disease infection on Block Island, Rhode Island. PLoS One 2014;9:e84758.
124. Phillips CB, Liang MH, Sangha O, et al. Lyme disease and preventive behaviors in residents of Nantucket Island, Massachusetts. Am J Prev Med 2001;20:219–24.
125. Vazquez M, Muehlenbein C, Cartter M, et al. Effectiveness of personal protective measures to prevent Lyme disease. Emerg Infect Dis 2008;14:210–6.
126. Aenishaenslin C, Michel P, Ravel A, et al. Factors associated with preventive behaviors regarding Lyme disease in Canada and Switzerland: a comparative study. BMC Public Health 2015;15:185.
127. Connally NP, Durante AJ, Yousey-Hindes KM, et al. Peridomestic Lyme disease prevention: results of a population-based case-control study. Am J Prev Med 2009;37:201–6.

Borrelia burgdorferi Pathogenesis and the Immune Response

 CrossMark

Mary Petzke, PhD, Ira Schwartz, PhD*

KEYWORDS

- Lyme disease • Genotypic variation • Adhesins • Type I interferon • Immune evasion

KEY POINTS

- *Borrelia burgdorferi* is highly invasive but does not produce any toxins. Lyme disease pathology is generally thought to be the result of host inflammatory response.
- There is substantial genotypic variation among *B burgdorferi* strains, and evidence suggests that certain strains have a greater probability of causing disseminated infection.
- *Borrelia burgdorferi* produces several adhesins that mediate binding to decorin, fibronectin, other glycosaminoglycans (GAGs), and integrins.
- Infection induces the synthesis of a variety of proinflammatory and antiinflammatory cytokines and chemokines by host immune cells that includes a type I interferon (IFNs) response that seems to depend on the genotype of the infecting *B burgdorferi* strain.
- The spirochete can evade the host immune response by resistance to complement-mediated killing facilitated by factor-H-binding proteins and by antigenic variation.

INTRODUCTION

Lyme disease, the most common vector-borne disease in North America and Europe,[1] is a multisystem disorder characterized by inflammation of affected tissues. Infection is initiated when spirochetes of the *B burgdorferi* sensu lato complex are deposited into the skin during the feeding of certain *Ixodes* ticks.[2] Some infections resolve at the site of inoculation, but if left untreated, skin-localized infection can progress to include distal target tissues following hematogenous dissemination of the spirochete.[3,4] The complex host-pathogen interactions that occur at the initial host-pathogen interface and determine the course of infection are likely influenced by multiple factors, including spirochete genotype, *B burgdorferi* proteins that mediate

Department of Microbiology and Immunology, New York Medical College, Valhalla, NY 10595, USA
* Corresponding author.
E-mail address: schwartz@nymc.edu

Clin Lab Med 35 (2015) 745–764
http://dx.doi.org/10.1016/j.cll.2015.07.004   labmed.theclinics.com

attachment and invasion, tick-derived components, host immune response, and *B burgdorferi* mechanisms of immune evasion. In this article, the authors review aspects of *B burgdorferi* pathogenesis and the host immune response to infection with regard primarily to *B burgdorferi* sensu stricto and host defenses at the initial host-pathogen interface in mammalian skin.

BORRELIA BURGDORFERI GENOMIC VARIATION

The genus *Borrelia* is composed of 2 major groups—the Lyme *Borrelia* and the relapsing fever *Borrelia*.[5] The Lyme *Borrelia* group contains 19 species, but only 4 (*B burgdorferi* sensu stricto, *Borrelia garinii*, *Borrelia afzelii*, and *Borrelia bavariensis*) cause human infection with any frequency.[5] In North America, the etiologic agent of virtually all Lyme disease is *B burgdorferi* sensu stricto (referred to hereinafter as *B burgdorferi*).

The *B burgdorferi* genome is unusual among bacteria in that it consists of multiple replicons. Whole genome sequencing of the type strain B31 revealed a 910-kb linear chromosome and 21 linear and circular plasmids.[6,7] Numerous studies involving a variety of molecular typing techniques established that there is substantial genotypic variation among *B burgdorferi* isolates.[8–14] This observation has been confirmed by whole genome sequencing of an additional 13 *B burgdorferi* isolates.[15] (It should be noted that as of this writing complete genome sequences, including all plasmids, are available for only 4 *B burgdorferi* strains—B31, N40, JD1, and ZS7; www. patricbrc.org). In addition to the chromosome, plasmids cp26 and lp54 and some cp32 replicons are present in all isolates.[13,16,17] The chromosome is essentially syntenic in all *B burgdorferi* strains except for minor variation at the right telomeric end, and the conserved portions are greater than 99% identical. The common 903-kb region of the chromosome encodes 815 putative open reading frames (ORFs) of greater than 50 amino acid residues and encompasses most of the housekeeping functions including metabolism, ion and nutrient transport, and information processing.[15,18]

By contrast, plasmid content among different *B burgdorferi* strains is quite heterogeneous, both with regard to the presence or absence of specific plasmid replicons and to sequence similarity[13,16,19]; this extensive heterogeneity has been confirmed by recent whole genome sequencing of multiple strains.[15,17] Plasmid content among 14 *B burgdorferi* isolates varied between 12 to 21 plasmids.[18] As a consequence, the putative number of ORFs varies from 1278 to 1521 among 4 fully sequenced *B burgdorferi* strains.[17]

Does this extensive genomic variation have implications for pathogenesis? The absence of certain plasmids results in reduced virulence in animal models of infection[20–23] or in ticks.[24–26] Wormser and colleagues,[27] using ribosomal spacer sequence typing, and Seinost and colleagues,[10] using outer surface protein C (OspC) typing, showed a significant association between the frequency of disseminated or invasive infection and certain *B burgdorferi* genotypes in patients with Lyme disease. This association was confirmed by subsequent studies with larger numbers of patients[28,29] and by multilocus sequence typing.[30] For example, a *B burgdorferi* genotype referred to as RST1/OspC type A was more frequently associated with disseminated infection in patients with Lyme disease.[10,27–29,31] The enhanced invasiveness of this genotype was confirmed in mouse infection studies.[32,33] More extensive whole genome sequencing of *B burgdorferi* isolates obtained from patients with Lyme disease is required to identify the genomic elements (genes, regulatory RNAs) that may be responsible for the variable pathogenic potential of different *B burgdorferi* genotypes.

BORRELIA BURGDORFERI PATHOGENIC MECHANISMS

Borrelia burgdorferi is a vector-borne pathogen that is deposited into mammalian skin by the bite of a tick vector.[2] The typical progression of a bacterial infection in a susceptible host involves adherence to the skin or mucosa, invasion and spread through blood or lymphatics, colonization of target tissue, and direct or indirect tissue damage by production of toxins or an induced inflammatory response. *Borrelia burgdorferi* is highly invasive, but there is no evidence that it produces any toxins; disease pathology is thought to result primarily from host inflammatory responses.[34,35] The best studied aspects of *B burgdorferi* pathogenesis are adhesion and immune evasion. Adaptation of *B burgdorferi* to its tick vector and mammalian host environments is also critical to its maintenance in nature and pathogenesis in disease-susceptible hosts. This process requires modulation of gene expression in these diverse milieus and is beyond the scope of this review. This aspect of *B burgdorferi* biology is the subject of several reviews and recent publications.[36–38] In this article, the authors focus on the *B burgdorferi* proteins that contribute directly to pathogenesis during mammalian infection.

BORRELIA BURGDORFERI ADHESINS

Numerous studies have shown that *B burgdorferi* can bind to a variety of cultured mammalian cells (reviewed in[39,40]). Subsequent investigations led to the identification of adhesins that are capable of mediating this interaction. Broadly, they can be classified into molecules that can bind to extracellular matrix (ECM) components and those that interact with integrins.[40]

Decorin Binding

Decorin is a small proteoglycan that associates with collagen and is a structural component of ECM. Infection of decorin-deficient mice with *B burgdorferi* resulted in lower bacterial burdens in skin and joints and reduced arthritis severity, suggesting a role for decorin binding in *B burgdorferi* pathogenesis.[41] *Borrelia burgdorferi* contains 2 decorin-binding proteins (Dbps), DbpA and DbpB, encoded in an operon on plasmid lp54.[6,7] These are 18- to 20-kDa surface-exposed lipoproteins that are only expressed during later stages of nymphal tick feeding and in the mammalian environment.[38,42] DbpA and DbpB are 41% identical at the amino acid level, but despite this similarity, they have somewhat distinctive GAG-binding specificities.[43] Several groups have generated *B burgdorferi* mutants lacking DbpA and DbpB and showed that the mutants are attenuated for mouse infection.[44–46] Surprisingly, transmission of DbpA/B-deficient mutants to mice via tick bite resulted in infection rates essentially indistinguishable from those of the wild-type strain.[44] The reason for the discrepancy between needle inoculation of in-vitro-grown spirochetes and tick-mediated infection is not known, but it may be the result of very low expression of *dbpA/B* during in vitro cultivation.[38,47,48] Taken together, the findings demonstrate that *B burgdorferi* binding to decorin is important for mammalian infection and that DpbA and DbpB are involved in the process.

Fibronectin Binding

Fibronectin is a glycoprotein component of the ECM that contains domains for interaction with heparin, collagen, and integrins.[49,50] Early studies showed that adherence of *B burgdorferi* to the ECM could be blocked by antibodies to fibronectin.[51] The best characterized *B burgdorferi* fibronectin-binding protein is BBK32, a plasmid-encoded 47-kDa protein.[52] Synthesis of BBK32 depends on the alternative sigma factor,

RpoS,[47] consistent with its elevated expression during mammalian infection.[53] Initial studies with BBK32-deficient mutants were contradictory. Seshu and colleagues[54] reported that these mutants were attenuated in experimental mouse infections, whereas Li and colleagues[55] demonstrated that BBK32 mutants retain full pathogenicity. More recent investigations using in vivo imaging approaches support a role for BBK32 during mouse infection,[56] perhaps by mediating vascular adhesion.[57] Interestingly, BBK32 also binds to GAGs, including heparin and dermatan sulfate.[58] Lin and colleagues[59] generated BBK32 mutants that were deficient in either fibronectin binding or GAG-binding capacity, demonstrating that these activities are mediated by 2 different functional domains. Furthermore, only GAG binding was required for joint colonization. These findings raise the possibility that GAG binding is the more critical function of BBK32 in mediating B burgdorferi infection.

Several other B burgdorferi proteins with fibronectin-binding activities have been described. Brissette and colleagues[60] demonstrated saturable binding of RevA, a 17-kDa protein encoded on a cp32 plasmid, to fibronectin. revA is expressed exclusively in mammalian tissue, but not in ticks.[38,60] A paralog of RevA, designated RevB, was also shown to bind fibronectin.[57,60] More recently, a chromosome-encoded protein, BB0347, was reported to be surface exposed and possess fibronectin-binding activity.[57,61] Moriarty and colleagues[57] reported that RevA, RevB, and BB0347 all bind fibronectin more weakly than BBK32 and that only BBK32 can restore vascular adhesion to a nonadhesive strain. However, vascular adhesion is reduced by only 20% in a BBK32-deficient mutant suggesting that other adhesins are required for this activity. It is possible that other proteins capable of interacting with GAGs (see below) also contribute to vascular adhesion.

Parveen and Leong[62] described a 26-kDa protein, encoded by the bb0588 chromosomal locus, that possesses GAG-binding activity and designated it Bgp. Curiously, Bgp also exhibits 5′-methyladenosine (MTA)/S-adenosyl homocysteine (SAH) nucleoside activity.[63] This enzyme removes MTA and SAH, toxic by-products produced during purine salvage or methionine metabolism. Infection of severe combined immunodeficiency (SCID) mice with a Bgp-deficient mutant was essentially indistinguishable from wild-type infection.[63] Borrelia burgdorferi contains a second protein with 5′-MTA/SAH nucleosidase activity and multiple other GAG-binding proteins. It is therefore possible that redundant activities of other proteins could replace those of Bgp during mammalian infection.

Integrin Binding

P66, a B burgdorferi protein encoded by the chromosomal locus bb0603, was initially identified as a channel-forming porin and was designated Oms66.[64,65] Subsequently, Coburn and colleagues[66] using phage display, identified P66 as a ligand for integrins $\alpha_{IIb}\beta_3$ and $\alpha_v\beta_3$ in vitro. Borrelia burgdorferi had previously been shown to bind $\alpha_{IIb}\beta_3$ and $\alpha_v\beta_3$ integrins,[67] and mutagenesis of bb0603 abrogated P66 conductance[65] and eliminated biding to $\alpha_v\beta_3$.[68] P66-deficient mutants are rapidly cleared from the site of inoculation in skin and cannot establish infection in either wild type, toll-like receptor 2 (TLR2)$^{-/-}$ or myeloid differentiation primary response gene 88 (MyD88)$^{-/-}$ mice, although they can survive in ticks.[69] More recent studies demonstrated that specific mutation of the integrin-binding domain of P66 did not affect infectivity of B burgdorferi delivered by subcutaneous inoculation, but infectivity was significantly reduced when B burgdorferi was delivered by intravenous inoculation. Furthermore, these site-directed mutants had reduced ability to cross an endothelial barrier.[70] The results suggest that P66 binding to β_3 integrins plays a role in B burgdorferi endothelial transmigration.

Behera and colleagues[71] identified BBB07, a protein encoded on cp26, as a ligand for integrin $\alpha_3\beta_1$. This protein is expressed during mammalian infection, and recombinant BBB07 induces interleukin (IL)-1β and IL-6 by cultured human chondrocytes. A definitive role for BBB07 in *B burgdorferi* pathogenesis awaits studies with BBB07-deficient spirochetes.

IMMUNE EVASION

The cell envelope of *B burgdorferi* is unusual in that it contains no lipopolysaccharide (LPS) as is the case for most proteobacteria, and instead contains a large number of lipoproteins.[6,72,73] *Borrelia burgdorferi* modulates lipoprotein expression under different environmental conditions and thereby alters its outer surface.[38] It is clear that numerous lipoproteins are expressed almost exclusively in either the mammalian or the tick vector.[38] It is reasonable to conclude that *B burgdorferi*'s ability to modify its outer surface by differential synthesis of lipoproteins could serve as an immune evasion process. However, the best studied immune evasion strategies used by *B burgdorferi* are antigenic variation and complement resistance.

Antigenic Variation

Borrelia burgdorferi strain B31 harbors a locus at the right telomeric end of plasmid lp28-1 that consists of a gene that encodes a 35-kDa lipoprotein designated VlsE and a series of 15 cassettes with extensive sequence similarity to VlsE. In a series of elegant experiments, Zhang and colleagues[74–76] showed that *vlsE* undergoes random segmented gene conversion whereby portions of the silent cassettes are substituted for sequences in the expressed *vlsE* resulting in a VlsE protein with substantial sequence variation. *vlsE* recombination does not occur during in vitro cultivation or in ticks.[76–78] In contrast, during infection of immunocompetent mice, recombination at the *vlsE* locus can be detected as early as 4 days postinfection and as many as 14 recombination events can be measured after 1 year of persistent infection. Although *vlsE* recombination also occurs in SCID mice, the number of recombination events is substantially reduced.[76,79]

Borrelia burgdorferi B31 derivatives lacking plasmid lp28-1 were severely attenuated in immunocompetent mice, but were capable of infecting and persisting in SCID mice.[20,21] Bankhead and Chaconas[80] constructed a *vlsE*-deficient strain and demonstrated that the *vlsE* locus was the region responsible for the lp28-1-deficient phenotype. Infection of SCID mice by *vlsE*-deficient mutants was indistinguishable from that of wild-type *B burgdorferi*.[80] The differences in the abilities of lp28-1- or *vlsE*-deficient strains to infect immunocompetent or SCID mice are consistent with the notion that VlsE antigenic variation is a major determinant for persistent *B burgdorferi* infection in mice. It should be noted that mice are natural reservoir hosts for *B burgdorferi* and remain persistently infected throughout their lifetimes. Although antibodies to VlsE are produced early during human Lyme disease, indicating that VlsE is expressed at this stage,[81] a role for VlsE in mediating persistent *B burgdorferi* infection in humans who have not been treated with a recommended regimen of antibiotics[3] remains to be clarified.

The detailed studies of lp28-1 and VlsE have virtually all been performed in the B31 strain background. Although some other *B burgdorferi* strains do not harbor an lp28-1-like plasmid, they do contain a *vls* locus on a different linear plasmid.[17] It is therefore reasonable to assume that the findings with strain B31 can be extended to other *B burgdorferi* strains.

Complement Resistance

The susceptibility of B burgdorferi sensu lato strains to complement-mediating killing varies.[82,83] Numerous investigators have demonstrated that this is due to the ability of these B burgdorferi strains to bind complement regulatory factor H or factor H-like protein-1.[83] Borrelia burgdorferi strains contain several factor H-binding proteins that interfere with the complement pathway by promoting inactivation of C3b[83,84]; B burgdorferi strain B31 encodes 5 such proteins. For simplicity, the foregoing discussion focuses on strain B31. Identical factor H-binding proteins have been given different designations based on either their function (eg, complement regulator acquiring surface protein [CRASP]) or their genetic locus.

CRASP-1 (CspA; BBA68) is a 29-kDa surface-exposed lipoprotein encoded by bba68 on plasmid lp54.[6,7] CRASP-1 binds factor H and factor H-like proteins.[84,85] Insertional inactivation of bba68 in a complement-resistant strain resulted in killing by human complement.[86] CRASP-1 is well expressed during the tick stages, but expression is strongly repressed during mammalian infection.[38,87,88] CRASP-2 (CspZ) is a 23-kDa lipoprotein encoded by bbh06 on plasmid lp28-3.[6,7] CRASP-2 binds factor H and factor H-like protein-1.[89] The expression pattern of CRASP-2 is essentially the mirror image of that of CRASP-1, being expressed during mammalian infection and at much lower levels in ticks.[38,88] Surprisingly, disruption of bbh06 did not result in complement sensitivity and the mutants were as infectious to mice as was the wild-type strain.[90] OspE, OspF, and Elp protein families (paralogous families 162, 163, 164[7]) comprise a group of lipoproteins encoded on cp32 plasmids. The proteins have extensive similarity, with some loci on distinct plasmids having identical sequences.[7] CRASP-3, 4, and 5 are also referred to as ErpP, ErpC, and ErpA/N, respectively; ErpP is encoded by bbn38, and ErpA is encoded by 3 separate loci on cp32-1, cp32-5, and cp32-8 (bbp38, bbl39). These proteins have high affinities for factor H.[83] Most members of the OspE/OspF/Elp families seem to be expressed during mammalian infection at levels greater than those expressed during tick colonization.[38,91] The redundancy of these proteins makes gene inactivation studies challenging, and so the roles of CRASP-3, 4, and 5 in infectivity and pathogenesis await further investigation.

BORRELIA BURGDORFERI VIRULENCE FACTORS

Numerous B burgdorferi genes/proteins have been described as having roles in maintenance of the spirochete in ticks or infectivity/pathogenesis in mammals (see Table 1 in[35] and Table 12.1 in[34]). In principle, all the proteins described in some detail in the preceding sections would qualify as virulence factors. In addition, several metabolic proteins (eg, PncA, AdeC, GuaA/B, GlpD, ChbC) have been shown to be required for maximal fitness in either a mammalian host or the tick vector.[23,92–98] Space does not permit an extensive discussion of all the potential virulence factors that have been identified. Here the authors describe the best studied B burgdorferi virulence factor, OspC.

OspC is the product of bbb19 (encoded on plasmid cp26).[6] OspC is not expressed in larvae or unfed nymphal ticks; its expression is induced during the nymphal blood meal and continues to increase during the early stages of mammalian infection.[38,99–102] Induction of ospC transcription depends on RpoS.[47,103] OspC-deficient strains are not infectious[104–106] because either they cannot migrate from the tick midgut to salivary glands or they cannot be transmitted during nymphal feeding.[104,105] OspC is required for establishment of infection, but its expression is repressed during persistent infection.[107–109] Repression seems to be mediated by

BBD18, a protein encoded on plasmid lp17.[110–112] Recently, Tilly and colleagues[113] showed that OspC is indeed required specifically during early infection, is downregulated, and is replaced by VlsE on the spirochetal surface during persistent infection. Despite intense investigation, the specific function of OspC is unclear. OspC can bind to a tick salivary gland protein, Salp15, which possesses immunomodulatory properties and may aid in *B burgdorferi* immune evasion during tick to mammal transmission.[114,115]

THE INNATE IMMUNE RESPONSE TO *BORRELIA BURGDORFERI*

The mammalian innate immune response provides an immediate reaction to a stimulus, such as an invading pathogen, that serves to control the threat until the development of an adaptive immune response is mounted. Components of the innate immune response include the complement system and specialized leukocytes. Species of *Borrelia* causing Lyme disease contain a variety of pathogen-associated molecular patterns (PAMPs) that are recognized by pattern recognition receptors (PRRs) expressed by cells of the mammalian immune system. TLRs, membrane-bound proteins located on the cell surface or within endosomal compartments, play a prominent role in the ligand-specific detection of *B burgdorferi* cellular components. Most TLRs use the adapter molecule MyD88 to initiate a signaling cascade that results in the production of cytokines and chemokines. Gram-negative bacteria are generally characterized by the presence of LPS, which initiates a robust inflammatory response through TLR4-dependent signaling. In contrast, as noted, *B burgdorferi* does not contain LPS, but instead expresses over 100 membrane-associated lipoproteins.[6,73] Most of these lipoproteins, including the abundant and well-characterized OspA and OspC, possess immunostimulatory properties conferred by the presence of a tripalmitoyl-S-glyceryl-cysteine (Pam$_3$Cys) modification.[116–121] Recognition of Pam$_3$Cys-modified *B burgdorferi* lipoproteins by TLR2 stimulates the nuclear translocation of nuclear factor-κB (NF-κB) and subsequent production of NF-κB-dependent cytokines (tumor necrosis factor [TNF], IL-6, IL-8) and adhesion factors (E-selectin, vascular cell adhesion molecule 1, and intracellular adhesion molecule 1) by human cell lines and/or human endothelial monolayers.[122–125] Consequently, activation of plasma-membrane-localized TLR2 by surface-exposed spirochetal lipoproteins was believed to be the primary pathway responsible for the expression of *Borrelia*-elicited cytokines and the induction of innate immunity. However, the existence of a TLR2-independent, but MyD88-dependent mechanism was implicated by the observation that *B burgdorferi*-infected TLR2-deficient mice displayed significantly greater inflammation in some infected tissues despite being unable to control spirochete burdens.[126,127] It is now well established that multiple PAMPs, PRRs, and signaling pathways contribute to the innate immune response to *B burgdorferi* in both humans and mice.

Maximal production of cytokines by human innate immune cells in response to *B burgdorferi* requires signaling from within the endolysosomal compartment following phagocytosis and spirochetal degradation.[128,129] In addition to contributing to the production of NF-κB-dependent cytokines, activation of endosomal TLR-dependent signaling pathways by bacterial nucleic acids is essential for the production of *Borrelia*-elicited type I IFNs (IFN-α and IFN-β) by human dendritic cells and monocytes.[130,131] TLR7 and TLR8 have recently been shown to recognize *B burgdorferi* RNA,[132,133] and TLR9 is an established receptor for nonmethylated CpG motifs of bacterial DNA.[134] *Borrelia burgdorferi* induces TLR7- and TLR9-mediated expression of IFN-α protein by human dendritic cells,[131] whereas transcriptional activation of

IFN-β is mediated by TLR8 in human monocytes.[135] Interaction between receptors has been documented, with cooperative signaling between TLR8 and TLR2 required for maximum production of the monocyte-derived cytokines TNF-α, IL-6, IL-10, and IL-1β.[135]

While the host-protective function of type I IFNs in antiviral defenses has been well established, the effects of type I IFNs with respect to bacterial infections are less well defined and seem to be highly variable.[136–140] Recently, TLR7- and TLR9-mediated signaling by human dendritic cells was also observed to promote *B burgdorferi*-induced secretion of type III IFN.[133] Similar to type I IFNs, type III IFNs have well-established roles in the antiviral response, but more recently identified and disparate effects with respect to bacterial pathogenesis.[141–144] The functions of these molecules in the host's response to *B burgdorferi* have not yet been elucidated. However, in ex vivo studies using human peripheral blood mononuclear cells, the induction of both IFN-α and IFN-λ1, a type III IFN, directly correlates with the pathogenic potential of the *B burgdorferi* genotype. Strains with greater capacity for dissemination from the skin induce significantly higher levels of these cytokines relative to strains that are attenuated for dissemination.[145]

THE INITIAL HOST-PATHOGEN INTERFACE: THE ERYTHEMA MIGRANS LESION

The complex interactions between the spirochete and the immune system of the mammalian host are initiated following deposition of the bacterium into the skin during tick feeding. Approximately 60% to 80% of human patients develop a primary erythema migrans (EM) skin lesion at the site of inoculation within 1 to 30 days after a tick bite.[4,146] EM is a localized immune response triggered by spirochete replication and migration through the skin. Despite the potential importance of immune interactions at the portal of entry, relatively few studies have investigated the immunopathogenesis of the EM lesion. Histopathological evaluation of punch biopsy specimens collected from the primary EM lesion of 42 Austrian patients with Lyme disease with presumed infection by *B afzelii* revealed a perivascular infiltrate of mononuclear cells composed predominantly of macrophages, T cells, and B cells, with a smaller number of plasma cells.[147] Examination of the EM biopsies using in situ hybridization with specific riboprobes identified the proinflammatory IFN-γ and the antiinflammatory IL-10 as the predominant cytokines expressed in the lesions. In addition, higher levels of the macrophage-derived proinflammatory cytokines, TNF-α, IL-1β, and IL-6, were expressed in the EM lesions of patients with systemic symptoms characteristic of disseminated disease.[147] A second study involving 128 Austrian patients infected with *B afzelii* detected elevated transcript levels for the T-cell-active chemokines, chemokine (C-X-C motif) ligand (CXCL) 9 and CXCL10, in the lesional skin along with lower but still significant mRNA levels for the neutrophil and dendritic cell chemoattractants, CXCL1 and chemokine (c-c motif) ligand (CCL) 20.[148] A more extensive analysis compared cytokine expression in EM lesions from *B afzelii*-infected Austrian patients and *B burgdorferi*-infected patients from the United States, all of whom had skin-culture-confirmed Lyme disease.[149] *Borrelia burgdorferi* elicited significantly higher mRNA levels for chemoattractants for neutrophils (CXCL1), macrophages (CCL3 and CCL4), and CD4+ T cells (CXCL9, CXCL10, CXCL11), in addition to higher mRNA expression of macrophage-associated proinflammatory cytokines IL-1β and TNF-α and antiinflammatory cytokines IL-10 and transforming growth factor. In addition, *B burgdorferi*-infected patients had faster-expanding lesions and more systemic symptoms when compared with *B afzelii*-infected patients.[149] The decreased induction of cytokines by *B afzelii* might underlie the observation that this species disseminates less frequently than *B burgdorferi* but is more likely to persist in the skin.[4,150]

The extent to which the nature and magnitude of the local immune response contributes to spirochetal containment or dissemination was the focus of a study involving 21 patients from the United States who were diagnosed with either skin-localized or disseminated *B burgdorferi* infection based on the presence of a single EM lesion or multiple EM lesions.[151] Epidermal suction blisters were raised over the periphery of the primary EM lesions, and cytokines and cell populations present in blister fluid aspirates were identified by multiparameter flow cytometry. Relative to the peripheral blood, EM blister fluids were enriched for $CD4^+$ and $CD8^+$ T cells, monocytes/macrophages, and both plasmacytoid and monocytoid dendritic cells, with a lower proportion of neutrophils.[151] Lesional innate immune mediators displayed enhanced expression of surface markers for activation and maturation, and the phenotype of T-cell subsets indicated that these cells were sensitized to *B burgdorferi* antigens. Flow cytometric analysis identified IL-6 and IFN-γ as the predominant cytokines present in EM blister fluids. Significantly higher levels of both of these proinflammatory cytokines, and significantly lower levels of antiinflammatory IL-10, were present in the EM blister fluids of patients with a single lesion compared with fluids of patients with multiple EM lesions.[151] This result suggests that a strong local IFN-γ-driven proinflammatory cytokine response during the early stages of infection contributes to host protection. In contrast, and consistent with ex vivo studies using human cells,[145] a potentially pathogen-promoting effect of type I IFN was implicated by the detection of significantly higher levels of IFN-α in blister fluids of patients with multiple EM lesions.[151]

EFFECT OF VECTOR-ENCODED FACTORS ON INNATE IMMUNITY

Studies focusing on vector-host interactions seem to support the correlation between inflammatory response and spirochete dissemination. Naturally acquired infections with Lyme-disease-causing *Borrelia* species are transmitted through the bite of an infected *Ixodes* tick and involve the deposition of tick salivary molecules into the skin. The immunomodulatory properties of tick saliva and subsequent effects on pathogen transmission at the cutaneous interface have been extensively reviewed.[152,153] Tick saliva and salivary proteins polarize the immune response toward an antiinflammatory profile primarily by suppressing multiple dendritic cell functions,[154] including $CD4^+$ T-cell proliferation[155] and differentiation,[156] spirochete phagocytosis,[155] and NF-κB-dependent signaling and cytokine production in response to stimulation by *Borrelia* or TLR agonists.[157,158] More recently, tick saliva, as well as a tick salivary cysteine protease inhibitor (sialostatin L2), was observed to interfere with type I IFN signaling via the Janus kinase/signal transducer and activator of transcription pathway in mouse dendritic cells, resulting in reduced expression of 2 IFN-stimulated genes, interferon regulatory factor-7 and interferon gamma-inducible protein-10.[159,160] However, it should be noted that *Borrelia*-induced levels of secreted IFN-β were not affected.[159] Coinoculation of *B burgdorferi* with *Ixodes scapularis* salivary gland lysate resulted in significantly higher spirochete burdens in the target tissues of needle-infected mice.[161] The immunosuppressive effects of tick saliva could be partially overcome by intraperitoneal administration of proinflammatory cytokines (IFN-γ, TNF-α, or IL-2, alone or in combination) for 10 days following tick infection with *B burgdorferi*; up to 95% protection was achieved, as determined by the presence of spirochetes or spirochetal DNA in ear tissues.[162] Similarly, spirochete burdens in infected tissues were significantly reduced following selective neutralization of 2 antiinflammatory cytokines, IL-4 and IL-5, in mice before transmission of B burgdorferi through tick feeding.[163]

CONCLUDING REMARKS

The mechanisms underlying B burgdorferi pathogenesis have been the subject of intensive study for over 25 years. Initially, these investigations were limited by the lack of robust tools for genetic manipulation of the spirochete. Since the introduction of these methods, much progress has been made in the elucidation of mechanisms for transcriptional regulation, adaptation to growth in the tick vector and mammalian host, host response, and immune evasion, but specific details of these processes remain to be clarified. Borrelia burgdorferi produces numerous adhesins with redundant functions; whether these proteins act at different stages of infection or in colonization of specific tissues is not yet known. Likewise, the roles of various lipoproteins in mediating complement resistance are not fully understood. With the application of newer technologies such as whole genome sequencing, transposon mutagenesis, and in vivo imaging, much progress in these and other aspects of B burgdorferi pathogenesis should be forthcoming in the near future.

SELF-ASSESSMENT

1. All of the following contribute to B burgdorferi pathogenesis except:
   A. Adhesion to ECM components
   B. Toxin production
   C. Induction of proinflammatory cytokines
   D. Evasion of the adaptive immune response
2. Genomic variation among B burgdorferi strains derives from:
   A. Deletions and insertion (indels) on the linear chromosome
   B. Rearrangements of chromosomal sequences
   C. Heterogeneity in plasmid content and sequence
   D. All of the above
3. Borrelia burgdorferi adhesins mediate interaction with target mammalian cells by binding to the following ECM components:
   A. Fibronectin
   B. Integrins
   C. Elastin
   D. Hyaluronic acid
4. TLR2 is the receptor for the following B burgdorferi cellular constituent:
   A. RNA
   B. Lipoproteins
   C. DNA
   D. LPS
5. Borrelia burgdorferi-induced production of type I IFN by human immune cells requires:
   A. Mast cell degranulation
   B. Generation of specific antibodies
   C. T-cell activation
   D. Phagocytosis

Answers
    Answer 1: B
    Answer 2: C
    Answer 3: A
    Answer 4: B
    Answer 5: D

REFERENCES

1. Mead PS. Epidemiology of Lyme disease. Infect Dis Clin North Am 2015;29: 187–210.
2. Ribeiro JM, Mather TN, Piesman J, et al. Dissemination and salivary delivery of Lyme disease spirochetes in vector ticks (Acari: Ixodidae). J Med Entomol 1987; 24:201–5.
3. Wormser GP, Dattwyler RJ, Shapiro ED, et al. The clinical assessment, treatment, and prevention of Lyme disease, human granulocytic anaplasmosis, and babesiosis: clinical practice guidelines by the Infectious Diseases Society of America. Clin Infect Dis 2006;43:1089–134.
4. Steere AC. Lyme disease. N Engl J Med 2001;345:115–25.
5. Wang G, Schwartz I. Genus Borrelia. In: Krieg NR, Parte A, Ludwig W, et al, editors. Bergey's manual of Systematic Bacteriology Volume four: the Bacteroidetes, Spirochaetes, Tenericutes (Mollicutes), Acidobacteria, Fibrobacteres, Fusobacteria, Dictyoglomi, Gemmatimonadetes, Lentisphaerae, Verrucomicrobia, Chlamydiae, and Planctomycetes, vol. 4, 2nd edition. New York: Springer; 2011. p. 484–531.
6. Fraser CM, Casjens S, Huang WM, et al. Genomic sequence of a Lyme disease spirochaete, *Borrelia burgdorferi*. Nature 1997;390:580–6.
7. Casjens S, Palmer N, van Vugt R, et al. A bacterial genome in flux: the twelve linear and nine circular extrachromosomal DNAs in an infectious isolate of the Lyme disease spirochete *Borrelia burgdorferi*. Mol Microbiol 2000;35:490–516.
8. Wang G, van Dam AP, Schwartz I, et al. Molecular typing of *Borrelia burgdorferi* sensu lato: taxonomic, epidemiological, and clinical implications. Clin Microbiol Rev 1999;12:633–53.
9. Liveris D, Gazumyan A, Schwartz I. Molecular typing of *Borrelia burgdorferi* sensu lato by PCR-restriction fragment length polymorphism analysis. J Clin Microbiol 1995;33:589–95.
10. Seinost G, Dykhuizen DE, Dattwyler RJ, et al. Four clones of *Borrelia burgdorferi* sensu stricto cause invasive infection in humans. Infect Immun 1999;67:3518–24.
11. Qiu WG, Schutzer SE, Bruno JF, et al. Genetic exchange and plasmid transfers in *Borrelia burgdorferi* sensu stricto revealed by three-way genome comparisons and multilocus sequence typing. Proc Natl Acad Sci U S A 2004;101:14150–5.
12. Bunikis J, Garpmo U, Tsao J, et al. Sequence typing reveals extensive strain diversity of the Lyme borreliosis agents *Borrelia burgdorferi* in North America and *Borrelia afzelii* in Europe. Microbiology 2004;150:1741–55.
13. Terekhova D, Iyer R, Wormser GP, et al. Comparative genome hybridization reveals substantial variation among clinical isolates of *Borrelia burgdorferi* sensu stricto with different pathogenic properties. J Bacteriol 2006;188:6124–34.
14. Margos G, Gatewood AG, Aanensen DM, et al. MLST of housekeeping genes captures geographic population structure and suggests a European origin of *Borrelia burgdorferi*. Proc Natl Acad Sci U S A 2008;105:8730–5.

15. Schutzer SE, Fraser-Liggett CM, Casjens SR, et al. Whole-genome sequences of thirteen isolates of *Borrelia burgdorferi*. J Bacteriol 2011;193:1018–20.

16. Iyer R, Kalu O, Purser J, et al. Linear and circular plasmid content in *Borrelia burgdorferi* clinical isolates. Infect Immun 2003;71:3699–706.

17. Casjens SR, Mongodin EF, Qiu WG, et al. Genome stability of Lyme disease spirochetes: comparative genomics of *Borrelia burgdorferi* plasmids. PLoS One 2012;7:e33280.

18. Mongodin EF, Casjens SR, Bruno JF, et al. Inter- and intra-specific pan-genomes of *Borrelia burgdorferi* sensu lato: genome stability and adaptive radiation. BMC Genomics 2013;14:693.

19. Palmer N, Fraser C, Casjens S. Distribution of twelve linear extrachromosomal DNAs in natural isolates of Lyme disease spirochetes. J Bacteriol 2000;182:2476–80.

20. Labandeira-Rey M, Skare JT. Decreased infectivity in *Borrelia burgdorferi* strain B31 is associated with loss of linear plasmid 25 or 28-1. Infect Immun 2001;69: 446–55.

21. Labandeira-Rey M, Seshu J, Skare JT. The absence of linear plasmid 25 or 28-1 of *Borrelia burgdorferi* dramatically alters the kinetics of experimental infection via distinct mechanisms. Infect Immun 2003;71:4608–13.

22. Purser JE, Norris SJ. Correlation between plasmid content and infectivity in *Borrelia burgdorferi*. Proc Natl Acad Sci U S A 2000;97:13865–70.

23. Purser JE, Lawrenz MB, Caimano MJ, et al. A plasmid-encoded nicotinamidase (PncA) is essential for infectivity of *Borrelia burgdorferi* in a mammalian host. Mol Microbiol 2003;48:753–64.

24. Strother KO, de Silva A. Role of *Borrelia burgdorferi* linear plasmid 25 in infection of *Ixodes scapularis* ticks. J Bacteriol 2005;187:5776–81.

25. Strother KO, Broadwater A, De Silva A. Plasmid requirements for infection of ticks by *Borrelia burgdorferi*. Vector Borne Zoonotic Dis 2005;5:237–45.

26. Grimm D, Tilly K, Bueschel DM, et al. Defining plasmids required by *Borrelia burgdorferi* for colonization of tick vector *Ixodes scapularis* (Acari: Ixodidae). J Med Entomol 2005;42:676–84.

27. Wormser GP, Liveris D, Nowakowski J, et al. Association of specific subtypes of *Borrelia burgdorferi* with hematogenous dissemination in early Lyme disease. J Infect Dis 1999;180:720–5.

28. Jones KL, Glickstein LJ, Damle N, et al. *Borrelia burgdorferi* genetic markers and disseminated disease in patients with early Lyme disease. J Clin Microbiol 2006;44:4407–13.

29. Wormser GP, Brisson D, Liveris D, et al. *Borrelia burgdorferi* genotype predicts the capacity for hematogenous dissemination during early Lyme disease. J Infect Dis 2008;198:1358–64.

30. Hanincova K, Mukherjee P, Ogden NH, et al. Multilocus sequence typing of *Borrelia burgdorferi* suggests existence of lineages with differential pathogenic properties in humans. PLoS One 2013;8:e73066.

31. Qiu WG, Bruno JF, McCaig WD, et al. Wide distribution of a high-virulence *Borrelia burgdorferi* clone in Europe and North America. Emerg Infect Dis 2008;14: 1097–104.

32. Wang G, Ojaimi C, Iyer R, et al. Impact of genotypic variation of *Borrelia burgdorferi* sensu stricto on kinetics of dissemination and severity of disease in C3H/HeJ mice. Infect Immun 2001;69:4303–12.

33. Wang G, Ojaimi C, Wu H, et al. Disease severity in a murine model of Lyme borreliosis is associated with the genotype of the infecting *Borrelia burgdorferi* sensu stricto strain. J Infect Dis 2002;186:782–91.

34. Norris SJ, Coburn J, Leong JM, et al. Pathobiology of Lyme disease *Borrelia*. In: Samuels DS, Radolf JD, editors. Borrelia: molecular biology, host interaction, and pathogenesis. Norfolk (United Kingdom): Caister Academic Press; 2010. p. 299–331.

35. Radolf JD, Caimano MJ, Stevenson B, et al. Of ticks, mice and men: understanding the dual-host lifestyle of Lyme disease spirochaetes. Nat Rev Microbiol 2012;10:87–99.

36. Skare JT, Carroll JA, Yang XF, et al. Gene regulation, transcriptomics, and proteomics. In: Samuels DS, Radolf JD, editors. Borrelia: molecular biology, host interaction, and pathogenesis. Norfolk (United Kingdom): Caister Academic Press; 2010. p. 67–101.

37. Samuels DS. Gene regulation in *Borrelia burgdorferi*. Annu Rev Microbiol 2011; 65:479–99.

38. Iyer R, Caimano MJ, Luthra A, et al. Stage-specific global alterations in the transcriptomes of Lyme disease spirochetes during tick feeding and following mammalian host adaptation. Mol Microbiol 2015;95:509–38.

39. Coburn J, Fischer JR, Leong JM. Solving a sticky problem: new genetic approaches to host cell adhesion by the Lyme disease spirochete. Mol Microbiol 2005;57:1182–95.

40. Antonara S, Ristow L, Coburn J. Adhesion mechanisms of *Borrelia burgdorferi*. Adv Exp Med Biol 2011;715:35–49.

41. Brown EL, Wooten RM, Johnson BJ, et al. Resistance to Lyme disease in decorin-deficient mice. J Clin Invest 2001;107:845–52.

42. Hagman KE, Yang X, Wikel SK, et al. Decorin-binding protein A (DbpA) of *Borrelia burgdorferi* is not protective when immunized mice are challenged via tick infestation and correlates with the lack of DbpA expression by B. burgdorferi in ticks. Infect Immun 2000;68:4759–64.

43. Groshong AM, Blevins JS. Insights into the biology of *Borrelia burgdorferi* gained through the application of molecular genetics. Adv Appl Microbiol 2014;86:41–143.

44. Blevins JS, Hagman KE, Norgard MV. Assessment of decorin-binding protein A to the infectivity of *Borrelia burgdorferi* in the murine models of needle and tick infection. BMC Microbiol 2008;8:82.

45. Shi Y, Xu Q, McShan K, et al. Both decorin-binding proteins A and B are critical for the overall virulence of *Borrelia burgdorferi*. Infect Immun 2008;76: 1239–46.

46. Weening EH, Parveen N, Trzeciakowski JP, et al. *Borrelia burgdorferi* lacking DbpBA exhibits an early survival defect during experimental infection. Infect Immun 2008;76:5694–705.

47. Caimano MJ, Iyer R, Eggers CH, et al. Analysis of the RpoS regulon in *Borrelia burgdorferi* in response to mammalian host signals provides insight into RpoS function during the enzootic cycle. Mol Microbiol 2007;65:1193–217.

48. Dunham-Ems SM, Caimano MJ, Eggers CH, et al. *Borrelia burgdorferi* requires the alternative sigma factor RpoS for dissemination within the vector during tick-to-mammal transmission. PLoS Pathog 2012;8:e1002532.

49. Singh P, Carraher C, Schwarzbauer JE. Assembly of fibronectin extracellular matrix. Annu Rev Cell Dev Biol 2010;26:397–419.

50. Henderson B, Nair S, Pallas J, et al. Fibronectin: a multidomain host adhesin targeted by bacterial fibronectin-binding proteins. FEMS Microbiol Rev 2011;35:147–200.

51. Szczepanski A, Furie MB, Benach JL, et al. Interaction between *Borrelia burgdorferi* and endothelium in vitro. J Clin Invest 1990;85:1637–47.

52. Probert WS, Johnson BJ. Identification of a 47 kDa fibronectin-binding protein expressed by *Borrelia burgdorferi* isolate B31. Mol Microbiol 1998;30:1003–15.

53. Fikrig E, Feng W, Barthold SW, et al. Arthropod- and host-specific *Borrelia burgdorferi bbk32* expression and the inhibition of spirochete transmission. J Immunol 2000;164:5344–51.

54. Seshu J, Esteve-Gassent MD, Labandeira-Rey M, et al. Inactivation of the fibronectin-binding adhesin gene *bbk32* significantly attenuates the infectivity potential of *Borrelia burgdorferi*. Mol Microbiol 2006;59:1591–601.

55. Li X, Liu X, Beck DS, et al. *Borrelia burgdorferi* lacking BBK32, a fibronectin-binding protein, retains full pathogenicity. Infect Immun 2006;74:3305–13.

56. Hyde JA, Weening EH, Chang M, et al. Bioluminescent imaging of *Borrelia burgdorferi* in vivo demonstrates that the fibronectin-binding protein BBK32 is required for optimal infectivity. Mol Microbiol 2011;82:99–113.

57. Moriarty TJ, Shi M, Lin YP, et al. Vascular binding of a pathogen under shear force through mechanistically distinct sequential interactions with host macromolecules. Mol Microbiol 2012;86:1116–31.

58. Fischer JR, LeBlanc KT, Leong JM. Fibronectin binding protein BBK32 of the Lyme disease spirochete promotes bacterial attachment to glycosaminoglycans. Infect Immun 2006;74:435–41.

59. Lin YP, Chen Q, Ritchie JA, et al. Glycosaminoglycan binding by *Borrelia burgdorferi* adhesin BBK32 specifically and uniquely promotes joint colonization. Cell Microbiol 2015;17:860–75.

60. Brissette CA, Bykowski T, Cooley AE, et al. *Borrelia burgdorferi* RevA antigen binds host fibronectin. Infect Immun 2009;77:2802–12.

61. Gaultney RA, Gonzalez T, Floden AM, et al. BB0347, from the Lyme disease spirochete *Borrelia burgdorferi*, is surface exposed and interacts with the CS1 heparin-binding domain of human fibronectin. PLoS One 2013;8:e75643.

62. Parveen N, Leong JM. Identification of a candidate glycosaminoglycan-binding adhesin of the Lyme disease spirochete *Borrelia burgdorferi*. Mol Microbiol 2000;35:1220–34.

63. Parveen N, Cornell KA, Bono JL, et al. Bgp, a secreted glycosaminoglycan-binding protein of *Borrelia burgdorferi* strain N40, displays nucleosidase activity and is not essential for infection of immunodeficient mice. Infect Immun 2006;74:3016–20.

64. Skare JT, Mirzabekov TA, Shang ES, et al. The Oms66 (p66) protein is a *Borrelia burgdorferi* porin. Infect Immun 1997;65:3654–61.

65. Pinne M, Thein M, Denker K, et al. Elimination of channel-forming activity by insertional inactivation of the *p66* gene in *Borrelia burgdorferi*. FEMS Microbiol Lett 2007;266:241–9.

66. Coburn J, Chege W, Magoun L, et al. Characterization of a candidate *Borrelia burgdorferi* beta3-chain integrin ligand identified using a phage display library. Mol Microbiol 1999;34:926–40.

67. Coburn J, Magoun L, Bodary SC, et al. Integrins alpha(v)beta3 and alpha5beta1 mediate attachment of Lyme disease spirochetes to human cells. Infect Immun 1998;66:1946–52.

68. Coburn J, Cugini C. Targeted mutation of the outer membrane protein P66 disrupts attachment of the Lyme disease agent, *Borrelia burgdorferi*, to integrin $a_V B_3$. Proc Natl Acad Sci U S A 2003;100:7301–6.

69. Ristow LC, Miller HE, Padmore LJ, et al. The b_3-integrin ligand of *Borrelia burgdorferi* is critical for infection of mice but not ticks. Mol Microbiol 2012;85:1105–18.

70. Ristow LC, Bonde M, Lin YP, et al. Integrin binding by *Borrelia burgdorferi* P66 facilitates dissemination but is not required for infectivity. Cell Microbiol 2015; 17(7):1021–36.
71. Behera AK, Durand E, Cugini C, et al. *Borrelia burgdorferi* BBB07 interaction with integrin a_3B_1 stimulates production of pro-inflammatory mediators in primary human chondrocytes. Cell Microbiol 2008;10:320–31.
72. Takayama K, Rothenberg RJ, Barbour AG. Absence of lipopolysaccharide in the Lyme disease spirochete, *Borrelia burgdorferi*. Infect Immun 1987;55:2311–3.
73. Setubal JC, Reis M, Matsunaga J, et al. Lipoprotein computational prediction in spirochaetal genomes. Microbiology 2006;152:113–21.
74. Zhang JR, Hardham JM, Barbour AG, et al. Antigenic variation in Lyme disease borreliae by promiscuous recombination of VMP-like sequence cassettes. Cell 1997;89:275–85.
75. Zhang JR, Norris SJ. Genetic variation of the *Borrelia burgdorferi* gene *vlsE* involves cassette-specific, segmental gene conversion. Infect Immun 1998;66:3698–704.
76. Zhang JR, Norris SJ. Kinetics and in vivo induction of genetic variation of *vlsE* in *Borrelia burgdorferi*. Infect Immun 1998;66:3689–97.
77. Indest KJ, Howell JK, Jacobs MB, et al. Analysis of *Borrelia burgdorferi vlsE* gene expression and recombination in the tick vector. Infect Immun 2001;69: 7083–90.
78. Ohnishi J, Schneider B, Messer WB, et al. Genetic variation at the *vlsE* locus of *Borrelia burgdorferi* within ticks and mice over the course of a single transmission cycle. J Bacteriol 2003;185:4432–41.
79. Coutte L, Botkin DJ, Gao L, et al. Detailed analysis of sequence changes occurring during *vlsE* antigenic variation in the mouse model of *Borrelia burgdorferi* infection. PLoS Pathog 2009;5:e1000293.
80. Bankhead T, Chaconas G. The role of VlsE antigenic variation in the Lyme disease spirochete: persistence through a mechanism that differs from other pathogens. Mol Microbiol 2007;65:1547–58.
81. Bacon RM, Biggerstaff BJ, Schriefer ME, et al. Serodiagnosis of Lyme disease by kinetic enzyme-linked immunosorbent assay using recombinant VlsE1 or peptide antigens of *Borrelia burgdorferi* compared with 2-tiered testing using whole-cell lysates. J Infect Dis 2003;187:1187–99.
82. Kurtenbach K, De Michelis S, Etti S, et al. Host association of *Borrelia burgdorferi* sensu lato–the key role of host complement. Trends Microbiol 2002;10:74–9.
83. Kraiczy P, Stevenson B. Complement regulator-acquiring surface proteins of *Borrelia burgdorferi*: structure, function and regulation of gene expression. Ticks Tick Borne Dis 2013;4:26–34.
84. Kraiczy P, Skerka C, Brade V, et al. Further characterization of complement regulator-acquiring surface proteins of *Borrelia burgdorferi*. Infect Immun 2001;69:7800–9.
85. Kraiczy P, Hellwage J, Skerka C, et al. Complement resistance of *Borrelia burgdorferi* correlates with the expression of BbCRASP-1, a novel linear plasmid-encoded surface protein that interacts with human factor H and FHL-1 and is unrelated to Erp proteins. J Biol Chem 2004;279:2421–9.
86. Brooks CS, Vuppala SR, Jett AM, et al. Complement regulator-acquiring surface protein 1 imparts resistance to human serum in *Borrelia burgdorferi*. J Immunol 2005;175:3299–308.
87. von Lackum K, Miller JC, Bykowski T, et al. *Borrelia burgdorferi* regulates expression of complement regulator-acquiring surface protein 1 during the mammal-tick infection cycle. Infect Immun 2005;73:7398–405.

88. Bykowski T, Woodman ME, Cooley AE, et al. Coordinated expression of *Borrelia burgdorferi* complement regulator-acquiring surface proteins during the Lyme disease spirochete's mammal-tick infection cycle. Infect Immun 2007;75: 4227–36.
89. Hartmann K, Corvey C, Skerka C, et al. Functional characterization of BbCRASP-2, a distinct outer membrane protein of *Borrelia burgdorferi* that binds host complement regulators factor H and FHL-1. Mol Microbiol 2006;61: 1220–36.
90. Coleman AS, Yang X, Kumar M, et al. *Borrelia burgdorferi* complement regulator-acquiring surface protein 2 does not contribute to complement resistance or host infectivity. PLoS One 2008;3:3010e.
91. Miller JC, von Lackum K, Babb K, et al. Temporal analysis of *Borrelia burgdorferi* Erp protein expression throughout the mammal-tick infectious cycle. Infect Immun 2003;71:6943–52.
92. Jewett MW, Lawrence K, Bestor AC, et al. The critical role of the linear plasmid lp36 in the infectious cycle of *Borrelia burgdorferi*. Mol Microbiol 2007;64:1358–74.
93. Jewett MW, Lawrence KA, Bestor A, et al. GuaA and GuaB are essential for *Borrelia burgdorferi* survival in the tick-mouse infection cycle. J Bacteriol 2009;191: 6231–41.
94. Margolis N, Hogan D, Tilly K, et al. Plasmid location of *Borrelia* purine biosynthesis gene homologs. J Bacteriol 1994;176:6427–32.
95. Zhou X, Cahoon M, Rosa P, et al. Expression, purification, and characterization of inosine 5'-monophosphate dehydrogenase from *Borrelia burgdorferi*. J Biol Chem 1997;272:21977–81.
96. Pappas CJ, Iyer R, Petze MM, et al. *Borrelia burgdorferi* requires glycerol for maximum fitness during the tick phase of the enzootic cycle. PLoS Pathog 2011;7:e1002102.
97. Tilly K, Elias AF, Errett J, et al. Genetics and regulation of chitobiose utilization in *Borrelia burgdorferi*. J Bacteriol 2001;183:5544–53.
98. Rhodes RG, Atoyan JA, Nelson DR. The chitobiose transporter, *chbC*, is required for chitin utilization in *Borrelia burgdorferi*. BMC Microbiol 2010;10:21.
99. Schwan TG, Piesman J, Golde WT, et al. Induction of an outer surface protein on *Borrelia burgdorferi* during tick feeding. Proc Natl Acad Sci U S A 1995;92: 2909–13.
100. Stevenson B, Schwan TG, Rosa PA. Temperature-related differential expression of antigens in the Lyme disease spirochete, *Borrelia burgdorferi*. Infect Immun 1995;63:4535–9.
101. Schwan TG, Piesman J. Temporal changes in outer surface proteins A and C of the Lyme disease-associated spirochete, *Borrelia burgdorferi*, during the chain of infection in ticks and mice. J Clin Microbiol 2000;38:382–8.
102. Mulay VB, Caimano MJ, Iyer R, et al. *Borrelia burgdorferi* bba74 is expressed exclusively during tick feeding and is regulated by both arthropod- and mammalian host-specific signals. J Bacteriol 2009;191:2783–94.
103. Hubner A, Yang X, Nolen DM, et al. Expression of *Borrelia burgdorferi* OspC and DbpA is controlled by a RpoN-RpoS regulatory pathway. Proc Natl Acad Sci U S A 2001;98:12724–9.
104. Grimm D, Tilly K, Byram R, et al. Outer-surface protein C of the Lyme disease spirochete: a protein induced in ticks for infection of mammals. Proc Natl Acad Sci U S A 2004;101:3142–7.
105. Pal U, Yang X, Chen M, et al. OspC facilitates *Borrelia burgdorferi* invasion of *Ixodes scapularis* salivary glands. J Clin Invest 2004;113:220–30.

106. Stewart PE, Wang X, Bueschel DM, et al. Delineating the requirement for the *Borrelia burgdorferi* virulence factor OspC in the mammalian host. Infect Immun 2006;74:3547–53.

107. Tilly K, Krum JG, Bestor A, et al. *Borrelia burgdorferi* OspC protein required exclusively in a crucial early stage of mammalian infection. Infect Immun 2006;74:3554–64.

108. Tilly K, Bestor A, Jewett MW, et al. Rapid clearance of Lyme disease spirochetes lacking OspC from skin. Infect Immun 2007;75:1517–9.

109. Xu Q, Seemanapalli SV, McShan K, et al. Constitutive expression of outer surface protein C diminishes the ability of *Borrelia burgdorferi* to evade specific humoral immunity. Infect Immun 2006;74:5177–84.

110. Sarkar A, Hayes BM, Dulebohn DP, et al. Regulation of the virulence determinant OspC by *bbd18* on linear plasmid lp17 of *Borrelia burgdorferi*. J Bacteriol 2011; 193:5365–73.

111. Casselli T, Tourand Y, Bankhead T. Altered murine tissue colonization by *Borrelia burgdorferi* following targeted deletion of linear plasmid 17-carried genes. Infect Immun 2012;80:1773–82.

112. Hayes BM, Dulebohn DP, Sarkar A, et al. Regulatory protein BBD18 of the Lyme disease spirochete: essential role during tick acquisition? MBio 2014;5: e01017–010114.

113. Tilly K, Bestor A, Rosa PA. Lipoprotein succession in *Borrelia burgdorferi*: similar but distinct roles for OspC and VlsE at different stages of mammalian infection. Mol Microbiol 2013;89:216–27.

114. Anguita J, Ramamoorthi N, Hovius JW, et al. Salp15, an *Ixodes scapularis* salivary protein, inhibits CD4(+) T cell activation. Immunity 2002;16:849–59.

115. Ramamoorthi N, Narasimhan S, Pal U, et al. The Lyme disease agent exploits a tick protein to infect the mammalian host. Nature 2005;436:573–7.

116. Brandt ME, Riley BS, Radolf JD, et al. Immunogenic integral membrane proteins of *Borrelia burgdorferi* are lipoproteins. Infect Immun 1990;58:983–91.

117. Radolf JD, Norgard MV, Brandt ME, et al. Lipoproteins of *Borrelia burgdorferi* and *Treponema pallidum* activate cachectin/tumor necrosis factor synthesis. Analysis using a CAT reporter construct. J Immunol 1991;147:1968–74.

118. Ma Y, Weis JJ. *Borrelia burgdorferi* outer surface lipoproteins OspA and OspB possess B-cell mitogenic and cytokine-stimulatory properties. Infect Immun 1993;61:3843–53.

119. Ma Y, Seiler KP, Tai KF, et al. Outer surface lipoproteins of *Borrelia burgdorferi* stimulate nitric oxide production by the cytokine-inducible pathway. Infect Immun 1994;62:3663–71.

120. Tai KF, Ma Y, Weis JJ. Normal human B lymphocytes and mononuclear cells respond to the mitogenic and cytokine-stimulatory activities of *Borrelia burgdorferi* and its lipoprotein OspA. Infect Immun 1994;62:520–8.

121. Radolf JD, Arndt LL, Akins DR, et al. *Treponema pallidum* and *Borrelia burgdorferi* lipoproteins and synthetic lipopeptides activate monocytes/macrophages. J Immunol 1995;154:2866–77.

122. Wooten RM, Modur VR, McIntyre TM, et al. *Borrelia burgdorferi* outer membrane protein A induces nuclear translocation of nuclear factor-kappa B and inflammatory activation in human endothelial cells. J Immunol 1996;157:4584–90.

123. Ebnet K, Brown KD, Siebenlist UK, et al. *Borrelia burgdorferi* activates nuclear factor-kappa B and is a potent inducer of chemokine and adhesion molecule gene expression in endothelial cells and fibroblasts. J Immunol 1997;158: 3285–92.

124. Hirschfeld M, Kirschning CJ, Schwandner R, et al. Cutting edge: inflammatory signaling by *Borrelia burgdorferi* lipoproteins is mediated by toll-like receptor 2. J Immunol 1999;163:2382–6.
125. Lien E, Sellati TJ, Yoshimura A, et al. Toll-like receptor 2 functions as a pattern recognition receptor for diverse bacterial products. J Biol Chem 1999;274: 33419–25.
126. Wooten RM, Ma Y, Yoder RA, et al. Toll-like receptor 2 is required for innate, but not acquired, host defense to *Borrelia burgdorferi*. J Immunol 2002;168: 348–55.
127. Wang G, Ma Y, Buyuk A, et al. Impaired host defense to infection and Toll-like receptor 2-independent killing of *Borrelia burgdorferi* clinical isolates in TLR2-deficient C3H/HeJ mice. FEMS Microbiol Lett 2004;231:219–25.
128. Moore MW, Cruz AR, LaVake CJ, et al. Phagocytosis of *Borrelia burgdorferi* and *Treponema pallidum* potentiates innate immune activation and induces gamma interferon production. Infect Immun 2007;75:2046–62.
129. Cruz AR, Moore MW, La Vake CJ, et al. Phagocytosis of *Borrelia burgdorferi*, the Lyme disease spirochete, potentiates innate immune activation and induces apoptosis in human monocytes. Infect Immun 2008;76:56–70.
130. Salazar JC, Duhham-Ems S, La Vake C, et al. Activation of human monocytes by live *Borrelia burgdorferi* generates TLR2-dependent and -independent responses which include induction of IFN-beta. PLoS Pathog 2009;5: e1000444.
131. Petzke MM, Brooks A, Krupna MA, et al. Recognition of *Borrelia burgdorferi*, the Lyme disease spirochete, by TLR7 and TLR9 induces a type I IFN response by human immune cells. J Immunol 2009;183:5279–92.
132. Cervantes JL, La Vake CJ, Weinerman B, et al. Human TLR8 is activated upon recognition of *Borrelia burgdorferi* RNA in the phagosome of human monocytes. J Leukoc Biol 2013;94:1231–41.
133. Love AC, Schwartz I, Petzke MM. *Borrelia burgdorferi* RNA induces type I and III interferons via Toll-like receptor 7 and contributes to production of NF-κB-dependent cytokines. Infect Immun 2014;82:2405–16.
134. Chuang TH, Lee J, Kline L, et al. Toll-like receptor 9 mediates CpG-DNA signaling. J Leukoc Biol 2002;71:538–44.
135. Cervantes JL, Dunham-Ems SM, La Vake CJ, et al. Phagosomal signaling by *Borrelia burgdorferi* in human monocytes involves Toll-like receptor (TLR) 2 and TLR8 cooperativity and TLR8-mediated induction of IFN-B. Proc Natl Acad Sci U S A 2011;108:3683–8.
136. Auerbuch V, Brockstedt DG, Meyer-Morse N, et al. Mice lacking the type I interferon receptor are resistant to *Listeria monocytogenes*. J Exp Med 2004;200: 527–33.
137. Carrero JA, Calderon B, Unanue ER. Type I interferon sensitizes lymphocytes to apoptosis and reduces resistance to *Listeria* infection. J Exp Med 2004;200: 535–40.
138. Mancuso G, Midiri A, Biondo C, et al. Type I IFN signaling is crucial for host resistance against different species of pathogenic bacteria. J Immunol 2007; 178:3126–33.
139. Mancuso G, Gambuzza M, Midiri A, et al. Bacterial recognition by TLR7 in the lysosomes of conventional dendritic cells. Nat Immunol 2009;10:587–94.
140. Parker D, Planet PJ, Soong G, et al. Induction of type I interferon signaling determines the relative pathogenicity of *Staphylococcus aureus* strains. PLoS Pathog 2014;10:e1003951.

141. Pietila TE, Latvala S, Osterlund P, et al. Inhibition of dynamin-dependent endocytosis interferes with type III IFN expression in bacteria-infected human monocyte-derived DCs. J Leukoc Biol 2010;88:665–74.
142. Lebreton A, Lakisic G, Job V, et al. A bacterial protein targets the BAHD1 chromatin complex to stimulate type III interferon response. Science 2011;331: 1319–21.
143. Bierne H, Travier L, Mahlakoiv T, et al. Activation of type III interferon genes by pathogenic bacteria in infected epithelial cells and mouse placenta. PLoS One 2012;7:e39080.
144. Cohen TS, Prince AS. Bacterial pathogens activate a common inflammatory pathway through IFNλ regulation of PDCD4. PLoS Pathog 2013;9:e1003682.
145. Krupna-Gaylord MA, Liveris D, Love AC, et al. Induction of type I and type III interferons by *Borrelia burgdorferi* correlates with pathogenesis and requires linear plasmid 36. PLoS One 2014;9:e100174.
146. Nadelman RB, Nowakowski J, Forseter G, et al. The clinical spectrum of early Lyme borreliosis in patients with culture-confirmed erythema migrans. Am J Med 1996;100:502–8.
147. Mullegger RR, McHugh G, Ruthazer R, et al. Differential expression of cytokine mRNA in skin specimens from patients with erythema migrans or acrodermatitis chronica atrophicans. J Invest Dermatol 2000;115:1115–23.
148. Mullegger RR, Means TK, Shin JJ, et al. Chemokine signatures in the skin disorders of Lyme borreliosis in Europe: predominance of CXCL9 and CXCL10 in erythema migrans and acrodermatitis and CXCL13 in lymphocytoma. Infect Immun 2007;75:4621–8.
149. Jones KL, Muellegger RR, Means TK, et al. Higher mRNA levels of chemokines and cytokines associated with macrophage activation in erythema migrans skin lesions in patients from the United States than in patients from Austria with Lyme borreliosis. Clin Infect Dis 2008;46:85–92.
150. Stanek G, Strle F. Lyme borreliosis. Lancet 2003;362:1639–47.
151. Salazar JC, Pope CD, Sellati TJ, et al. Coevolution of markers of innate and adaptive immunity in skin and peripheral blood of patients with erythema migrans. J Immunol 2003;171:2660–70.
152. Kazimirova M, Stibraniova I. Tick salivary compounds: their role in modulation of host defences and pathogen transmission. Front Cell Infect Microbiol 2013;3:43.
153. Wikel S. Ticks and tick-borne pathogens at the cutaneous interface: host defenses, tick countermeasures, and a suitable environment for pathogen establishment. Front Microbiol 2013;4:337.
154. Mason LM, Veerman CC, Geijtenbeek TB, et al. Menage a trois: Borrelia, dendritic cells, and tick saliva interactions. Trends Parasitol 2014;30:95–103.
155. Slamova M, Skallova A, Palenikova J, et al. Effect of tick saliva on immune interactions between *Borrelia afzelii* and murine dendritic cells. Parasite Immunol 2011;33:654–60.
156. Mejri N, Brossard M. Splenic dendritic cells pulsed with *Ixodes ricinus* tick saliva prime naive CD4+T to induce Th2 cell differentiation in vitro and in vivo. Int Immunol 2007;19:535–43.
157. Hovius JW, de Jong MA, den Dunnen J, et al. Salp15 binding to DC-SIGN inhibits cytokine expression by impairing both nucleosome remodeling and mRNA stabilization. PLoS Pathog 2008;4:e31.
158. Lieskovska J, Kopecky J. Effect of tick saliva on signalling pathways activated by TLR-2 ligand and *Borrelia afzelii* in dendritic cells. Parasite Immunol 2012; 34:421–9.

159. Lieskovska J, Kopecky J. Tick saliva suppresses IFN signalling in dendritic cells upon *Borrelia afzelii* infection. Parasite Immunol 2012;34:32–9.
160. Lieskovska J, Palenikova J, Sirmarova J, et al. Tick salivary cystatin sialostatin L2 suppresses IFN responses in mouse dendritic cells. Parasite Immunol 2015;37:70–8.
161. Zeidner NS, Schneider BS, Nuncio MS, et al. Coinoculation of *Borrelia spp.* with tick salivary gland lysate enhances spirochete load in mice and is tick species-specific. J Parasitol 2002;88:1276–8.
162. Zeidner N, Dreitz M, Belasco D, et al. Suppression of acute Ixodes scapularis-induced *Borrelia burgdorferi* infection using tumor necrosis factor-alpha, interleukin-2, and interferon-gamma. J Infect Dis 1996;173:187–95.
163. Zeidner NS, Schneider BS, Rutherford JS, et al. Suppression of Th2 cytokines reduces tick-transmitted *Borrelia burgdorferi* load in mice. J Parasitol 2008;94: 767–9.

Clinical Manifestations and Treatment of Lyme Disease

Joyce L. Sanchez, MD

KEYWORDS

- Lyme disease • *Borrelia burgdorferi* • Lyme disease treatment
- Post-Lyme disease syndrome

KEY POINTS

- Early, disseminated infection can present as a flulike illness, as disseminated erythema migrans, or with more serious neurologic or cardiac complications.
- Late infection can result in inflammatory oligoarticular arthritis requiring a longer course of antibiotics.
- For early infection, oral doxycycline for 14 to 21 days is recommended.
- For inflammatory arthritis or active neurologic disease, longer courses of oral doxycycline or intravenous ceftriaxone for 28 days may be necessary.
- Continued symptoms despite antibiotic therapy should be treated symptomatically and sometimes require a multidisciplinary approach, with consideration of treating other comorbid conditions.

INTRODUCTION

More than 27,000 confirmed cases of Lyme disease were reported in 2013, making it the most common tick-borne disease in the United States.[1] It is also found in parts of both Europe and Asia. The causative agents of Lyme disease include *Borrelia burgdorferi* in the United States and *Borrelia afzelii* and *Borrelia garinii* in Europe, which are transmitted to humans by *Ixodes* species ticks. Cases are seen more frequently during the spring, summer, and early fall months. The clinical manifestations of infection can vary, ranging from a local skin reaction, to systemic syndromes, and dissemination to other organ systems including the joints, heart, and central nervous system.

Disclosure Statement: The author has nothing to disclose.
Division of General Internal Medicine, Mayo Clinic, 200 First Street Southwest, Rochester, MN 55905, USA
E-mail address: sanchez.joyce@mayo.edu

Clin Lab Med 35 (2015) 765–778
http://dx.doi.org/10.1016/j.cll.2015.08.004
0272-2712/15/$ – see front matter © 2015 Elsevier Inc. All rights reserved.

NATURAL COURSE OF UNTREATED DISEASE

The incubation period between infection and initial clinical manifestations is generally between 7 and 14 days, although in some cases symptom onset has been documented to range from 3 to 30 days after exposure. Asymptomatic infection with spontaneous clearance is unusual but has been noted to occur in 10% of individuals in the United States.[2] Steere[3] has defined and described the stages of Lyme disease following symptom onset, which are reviewed in the later sections (**Fig. 1**, **Table 1**).

EARLY, LOCALIZED LYME DISEASE

In early, localized disease (stage 1), the classic initial manifestation is erythema migrans, also known as a "bull's-eye rash," typically appearing at the site of tick attachment (see **Fig. 1**). The diagnosis of erythema migrans is made based on the patient's history, including tick exposure in a Lyme endemic area, and physical examination. The lesion is pathognomonic for Lyme disease, and serologic testing is not recommended to confirm the diagnosis at this stage. The rash begins as a painless, nonpruritic, red papule that expands to a red annular lesion measuring 5 to 30 cm in diameter. In some cases, however, the central red papule may appear necrotic or vesicular.[4,5] Although there may be some central clearing resulting in the bull's-eye appearance, many lesions have uniform erythema throughout, and repeat infections may present with or without central clearing of the erythema migrans rash. Notably, up to 20% of patients may not develop or do not recall an erythema migrans rash.[6] Other associated symptoms indicative of the inflammatory response to early infection include fever, malaise, and regional lymphadenopathy. Erythema migrans lesions can persist for a few days and up to 3 to 4 weeks.[7] In Europe, B afzelli and B garinii can present with lymphocytoma, a firm, colored, painless, nodular lesion most commonly found around the earlobes or nipples (**Fig. 2**).

EARLY DISSEMINATED LYME DISEASE

In early, disseminated disease (stage 2), often occurring in the absence of initial treatment, Borrelia will spread hematogenously from the initial site of infection to other organ systems. Over the course of days to weeks, secondary annual lesions with similar appearance to the first erythema migrans lesion may appear throughout the body, indicating dissemination. Less typical skin eruptions include a malar rash of the face

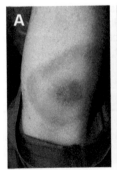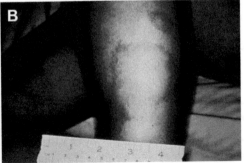

Fig. 1. (A) Erythema migrans of localized Lyme disease and (B) multiple erythema migrans lesions in disseminated disease. (Courtesy of The Center for Disease Control and Prevention's Public Health Image Library [Identification numbers 9875 and 14475].)

Table 1
Stages and clinical manifestations of Lyme disease

System	Early Infection		Late Infection
	Localized Stage 1	Disseminated Stage 2	Persistent Stage 3
Skin	Erythema migrans	Secondary annular lesions Malar rash Diffuse erythema or urticaria Evanescent lesions Lymphocytoma	Acrodermatitis chronica atrophicans Localized scleroderma-like lesions
Musculoskeletal	—	Migratory pain in joints, tendons, bursae, muscle, bone Brief arthritis attacks Myositis[a] Osteomyelitis[a] Panniculitis[a]	Prolonged arthritis attacks Chronic arthritis Peripheral enthesopathy Periostitis or joint subluxations below acrodermatitis
Neurologic	—	Meningitis Cranial neuritis, facial palsy Motor or sensory radiculoneuritis Subtle encephalitis Mononeuritis multiplex Pseudotumor cerebri Myelitis[a] Cerebellar ataxia[a]	Chronic encephalomyelitis Spastic paraparesis Ataxic gait Subtle mental disorders Chronic axonal polyradiculopathy
Lymphatic	Regional lymphadenopathy	Regional or generalized lymphadenopathy Splenomegaly	—
Heart	—	AV nodal block Myopericarditis Pancarditis	—
Eyes	—	Conjunctivitis Iritis[a] Choroiditis[a] Retinal hemorrhage or detachment[a] Panophthalmitis[a]	Keratitis
Liver	—	Mild or recurrent hepatitis	—
Respiratory	—	Nonexudative sore throat Nonproductive cough	—
Kidney	—	Microscopic hematuria or proteinuria	—
Genitourinary	—	Orchitis[a]	—
Constitutional systems	Minor	Severe malaise and fatigue	Fatigue

[a] Should be considered possible but not proven manifestations of Lyme disease.
From Steere AC. Lyme disease. N Engl J Med 1989;321(9):586; with permission.

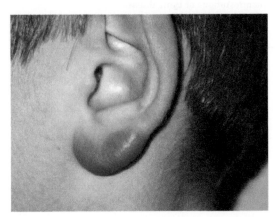

Fig. 2. Lymphocytoma of the ear due to *Borrelia* infection. (*From* Palmen C, Jamblin P, Flor-kin B, et al. Borrelia-associated lymphocytoma cutis. Arch Pediatr 2010;8:1160; with permission.)

and a diffuse erythematous or urticarial rash. Patients often experience fever, chills, malaise, fatigue, headache, arthralgia, myalgia, lymphadenopathy, and neck and joint stiffness. These symptoms may be continuous or intermittent. Neurologic signs include cranial neuropathies. Facial palsy or Bell's palsy is the most common cranial neuropathy and can be either unilateral or bilateral (**Fig. 3**). Motor or sensory radicu-lopathies have also been described. These neurologic manifestations have been

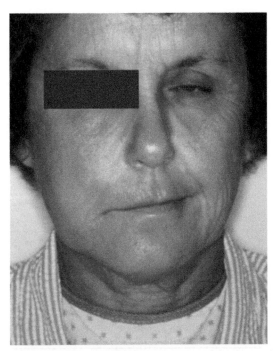

Fig. 3. Facial palsy in disseminated Lyme disease. (*Courtesy of* the Center for Disease Control and Prevention's Public Health Image Library [Identification number 6633].)

seen in approximately 15% of untreated patients in the United States.[8] A more detailed discussion of neurologic symptoms can be found in the article by Halperin of this issue.[9] Ocular manifestations are rare but have been reported in association with Lyme disease and are listed in **Table 1**.

Less common manifestations during this stage include lymphocytic meningitis, encephalitis, and cerebral ataxia. Several case reports have suggested that Lyme disease can be implicated as a source for sudden sensorineural hearing loss, especially when associated with other symptoms consistent with Lyme disease (recent erythema migrans, for example) or a positive serology.[10] Cardiovascular abnormalities may also occur and affect approximately 4% to 8% of untreated patients. Acute atrioventricular (AV) block is the most common cardiac conduction abnormality, which may present with dizziness, light-headedness, or syncope, or may be asymptomatic. Myopericarditis, or Lyme carditis, can present with chest pain, dyspnea, or syncope.[11]

LATE LYME DISEASE

Late, persistent Lyme disease (stage 3) most often presents as inflammatory oligoarticular arthritis several months after the initial infection and has been reported to occur in approximately 11% of patients with untreated erythema migrans. The arthritis is generally asymmetric and affects the large, weight-bearing joints, particularly the knees (**Fig. 4**). Symptoms can range in presentation from mild and intermittent pain to severe and erosive disease.[12] Analysis of synovial fluid aspirated from the affected joint demonstrates an inflammatory arthritis with elevated leukocyte counts of approximately 25,000/mm^3, with a polymorphonucleocyte predominance. Although most patients will respond to and have resolution of their arthritic symptoms following antibiotic therapy, a subset may continue to have persistent inflammatory arthritis referred to as antibiotic-refractory Lyme arthritis. Both organism-specific and host factors are thought to play a role in these cases. Certain strains, more commonly found in the Northeast Unites States, are more virulent and associated with higher levels inflammatory cytokines (tumor necrosis factor-α and interferon-γ) in synovial fluid. Host factors include patients with certain HLA-DR alleles and TLR1 polymorphisms.[13]

Chronic skin lesions of achrodermatitis chronica can be seen in Asia and Europe with *B afzelii* infection.[14,15] This condition begins with mild inflammatory lesions of the extensor surfaces of the limbs, which progress to more violaceous lesions that eventually lead to skin atrophy (**Fig. 5**).

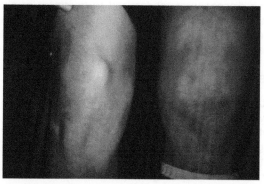

Fig. 4. Inflammatory arthritis in late Lyme disease. (*Courtesy of* The Center for Disease Control and Prevention's Public Health Image Library [Identification number 14472].)

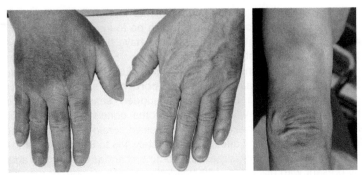

Fig. 5. Achrodermatitis chronica due to *Borrelia* infection. (*From* Zajkowska J, Czupryna P, Pancewicz SA, et al. Acrodermatitis chronica atrophicans. Lancet Infect Dis 2011;11:800; with permission.)

POST-LYME DISEASE SYMPTOMS

After appropriate antibiotic therapy for Lyme disease, 10% to 20% of patients may continue to experience mild symptoms for several weeks, and up to 6 months, which many be referred to as post-Lyme disease symptoms.[16] These symptoms most commonly include fatigue, arthralgia, myalgia, and mild cognitive complaints. The symptoms are ultimately self-limited and resolve without further treatment. The cause for persistence of these symptoms is not entirely understood; however, comorbid conditions and external stressors may play a role.

POST-LYME DISEASE SYNDROME

Nevertheless, a smaller subset of patients continue to have the symptoms described for 6 months or longer; this condition is referred to as post-Lyme disease syndrome. Some patients and medical groups, including the International Lyme and Associated Diseases Society, define this illness as chronic Lyme disease and think that the cause is due to persistent infection with *B burgdorferi*, ultimately requiring prolonged antibiotic therapy. Importantly, however, there are no replicated studies demonstrating persistent infection with *B burgdorferi* following appropriate antibiotic treatment.[16] Furthermore, several randomized controlled trials have demonstrated no improvement in symptoms after prolonged courses of antibiotics.[17–19] In one study, patients with musculoskeletal pain, neurocognitive symptoms, and fatigue persisting after well-documented, previously treated Lyme disease were randomized to treatment or placebo. Treatment included prolonged intravenous (IV) ceftriaxone and oral doxycycline for 90 days. No difference was seen in scales measuring the health-related quality of life, and the study was stopped because of the lack of significant improvement in the treatment arm.

CONGENITAL INFECTION

Congenitally acquired Lyme disease is extremely rare. Stillbirth and congenital heart abnormalities have been described; however, definitive evidence of *B burgdorferi* infection of the fetus has not been shown.[20–23] A review of 95 women who presented with erythema migrans during pregnancy in Budapest and Hungary, Lakos and Solymosi[24] documented an increase in adverse pregnancy outcomes, including pregnancy loss and cavernous hemangioma, which was statistically significant in mothers who had not received antibiotic therapy compared with those who had completed an appropriate course.

RELAPSE VERSUS REINFECTION

Concern has been raised regarding the question of relapsing Lyme disease. Studies of patients who experience more than one episode of documented Lyme disease have shown that repeated episodes of erythema migrans are due to reinfections rather than a relapse of a prior infection.[25] This finding is not surprising given the risk of re-exposure to *Ixodes* ticks with every season in patients who live in endemic areas. Treatment of early reinfection is the same as the initial infection (see Therapy section).

DIFFERENTIAL DIAGNOSIS

Erythema migrans is diagnosed with a careful physical examination and review of patient history, including the risk of tick exposure and outdoor activity in a Lyme endemic area. Although pathognomonic for Lyme disease, several other entities may be mistaken for erythema migrans and should be considered in patients, especially if the time of year or geography makes Lyme disease unlikely.[7] In the southeastern and south central United States, southern tick-associated rash illness (STARI) can present with a lesion very similar to the one associated with Lyme disease. Although the cause is not fully understood, and diagnostic testing for STARI is not currently available, there are no other clinical manifestations (eg, myalgia, arthralgia, fever) of the disease. Other potential mimics of erythema migrans include hypersensitivity response to a tick or other insect bites, which typically result in a pruritic response, with small, raised centers. Spider bites, which can present with a painful, necrotic skin lesion with central necrosis, may also be misidentified as erythema migrans. For patients with a rapidly enlarging lesion of erythema and pain, one must consider cellulitis, which can be superimposed on a bite or other site of trauma. Tinea can present with a rash with raised margins and central clearing and is generally pruritic. Nummular eczema and granuloma annulare can also be mistaken for erythema migrans; however, these lesions are usually small and do not rapidly enlarge. Erythema multiforme can appear similar to multiple erythema migrans lesions, but a distinguishing feature is the involvement of the palms and soles.[7,26]

Neurologic symptoms, including cranial nerve palsies, are often seen with viral infections such as herpes simplex virus. Less common infections that have been implicated in facial palsies include cytomegalovirus, Epstein-Barr virus, adenovirus, rubella virus, mumps, influenza B, and coxsackievirus.[27] Otitis media, which on rare occasions can present with facial palsy, can be excluded with examination of the middle ear. It is also generally recommended that patients with unexplained neurologic symptoms be evaluated for both human immunodeficiency virus and syphilis, particularly if there are any risk factors.

With respect to patients with arthritic symptoms, for active patients presenting with monoarticular joint pain, especially of the knee, mechanical injury should be considered and ruled out before rigorous evaluation for Lyme disease. For young individuals with oligoarticular arthritis, the possibility of juvenile rheumatoid arthritis should be evaluated. Seronegative spondyloarthropathies, including ankylosing spondylitis, reactive arthritis, and psoriatic arthritis, can affect the large joints in an asymmetric manner. In patients with multiple somatic symptoms and prolonged fatigue and myalgia, fibromyalgia and chronic fatigue syndrome should also be considered.

THERAPY

The latest guidelines from the Infectious Disease Society of America (IDSA) for the treatment of Lyme disease were released in 2006.[28] A more comprehensive guideline on the prevention, diagnosis, and treatment of Lyme disease is being developed and reviewed regularly by the IDSA in collaboration with the American Academy of Neurology and the American College of Rheumatology. Groups including the American Academy of Neurology and other professional societies in Europe have also released similar treatment guidelines. In general, B burgdorferi commonly demonstrates susceptibility in vitro to macrolides, penicillins, and third-generation cephalosporins, with inherent resistance to quinolones, rifampin, and aminoglycosides.[28,29] The following section reviews appropriate treatment regimens for the various clinical manifestations of Lyme disease.

EARLY INFECTION

The mainstay of treatment of early Lyme disease, both localized and disseminated, is oral doxycycline (refer to **Table 2** for detailed dosing recommendations). Treatment of children and during pregnancy is described later. For individuals in whom doxycycline is contraindicated, viable alternatives include amoxicillin and cefuroxime. Complete resolution of all symptoms with any of these 3 drugs approaches 90%. Macrolides, while active against B burgdorferi in vitro, should be considered a distant alternative for patient management. Cure rates are significantly lower, approximately 80%.[28] Randomized

Table 2
Lyme disease treatment

Early Infection	Treatment and Dosing Regimen
Adults	Doxycycline, 100 mg orally twice a day for 14–21 days OR Amoxicillin, 500 mg orally 3 times a day for 14–21 days (can be used in pregnancy) *Alternative:* Cefuroxime axetil, 500 mg orally twice a day for 14–21 days
Children (age 8 or younger)	Amoxicillin 50 mg/kg/day orally, divided into three doses per day for 14–21 days *Alternative:* Cefuroxime axetil 30 mg/kg/day orally, divided into two doses per day for 14–21 days
Neurologic abnormalities	—
Adults	Ceftriaxone, 2 g IV once a day for 14–28 days OR Cefotaxime 6 g/day IV, divided into doses every 8 hours *Alternative:* Doxycycline, 100 mg orally 3 times a day for 14–28 days
Children	Ceftriaxone 50–75 mg/kg/d IV daily for 14–28 days OR Cefotaxime 150–200 mg/kg/d IV, divided into doses every 8 hours
Cranial nerve palsy alone	Same as early infection
Carditis	—
First-degree AV block (P-R interval >0.3 s)	Oral regimens, as for early infection
High-degree AV block	Ceftriaxone, 2 g IV once a day for 14–21 days, treatment may be completed with an oral agent
Arthritis	Same doses for oral and parenteral agents for 28 days. For persistent symptoms, a second course of oral agents or a 14–28-day course of parenteral agents can be used

Adapted from Shapiro ED. Clinical practice. Lyme disease. N Engl J Med 2014;370(18):1729; with permission.

controlled trials comparing a 10- to 14-day course of doxycycline versus a 21-day course, or compared with IV ceftriaxone, have found no significant differences in cure rates.[30,31] Finally, approximately 15% of patients will experience initial exacerbation of their symptoms within 24 hours after treatment; this is referred to as the Jarisch-Herxheimer reaction and is largely due to the lysis of spirochetes. These symptoms resolve within 48 hours of onset without the need for additional or alternative treatment.

Symptomatic patients with carditis, or those who are found to have AV nodal block, should be hospitalized and monitored while receiving parenteral antibiotics, usually ceftriaxone. Therapy with antiarrhythmics or a pacemaker may be needed for advanced AV nodal block. Once discharged, the patient may be asked to complete a 14- to 28-day course with oral antibiotics.

Individuals with evidence of active central nervous system disease (eg, meningitis, acute radiculopathy) and objective neurologic findings are also treated with a 14- to 28-day course of IV ceftriaxone. A notable exception to this practice is treatment of isolated facial palsy with a course of oral doxycycline for 14 to 21 days. Data supporting this practice have largely arisen from numerous European studies, which indicate that individuals (children and adults) with acute neuroborreliosis who received oral doxycycline had equivalent recovery compared with individuals who received IV penicillin or ceftriaxone therapy.[32,33]

LATE INFECTION

Patients with late Lyme disease, including inflammatory arthritis, should be treated with oral doxycycline (or another oral alternative) for 4 to 8 weeks. Adjunctive treatment with nonsteroidal anti-inflammatory drugs is also useful. For cases of persistent or recurring arthritis, a second course of oral antibiotics or parenteral treatment may be considered.

TREATMENT OF CHILDREN AND DURING PREGNANCY

Pregnant women and children should be treated according to their stage of disease. For children greater than 8 years of age, oral doxycycline can be used. In those age 8 or younger, amoxicillin is the preferred oral agent, with cefuroxime or erythromycin as alternatives. Doxycycline should be avoided in pregnancy; oral alternatives include amoxicillin and cefuroxime.

POST-LYME DISEASE SYMPTOMS/SYNDROME

As indicated above, several randomized controlled trials have demonstrated no improvement in post-Lyme disease syndrome following prolonged courses of IV antibiotics.[17–19] In addition, the extended duration of IV antibiotics has been associated with significant sequelae, unrelated to Lyme disease. Antibiotics such as ceftriaxone carry the risk of cholestasis requiring cholecystectomy, and indwelling venous catheters carry the risk of bloodstream infection and deep venous thrombosis. Many patients on prolonged antibiotic courses may develop severe gastrointestinal disease due to *Clostridium difficile*. Although rare, death due to the complications associated with long-term treatment of Lyme disease, although not directly associated with the initial *B burgdorferi* infection, have also been reported. Finally, it is worthwhile to note that identifying patients who meet the inclusion criteria for post-Lyme disease syndrome, which includes documented evidence of prior Lyme disease and ongoing symptoms despite treatment, is challenging. In and of itself, this demonstrates the paucity of patients with objective Lyme disease who have chronic symptoms after initial treatment.

Although anecdotal evidence among individuals with post-Lyme disease syndrome shows trends toward symptom improvement with antibiotics, several pitfalls existed with these studies.[34–36] These limitations include using loose case definitions for post-Lyme disease syndrome and interpretation of Lyme disease diagnostic testing criteria that is not consistent with the current recommendations by the Centers for Disease Control and Prevention. In addition, controlled trials found that up to 40% of subjects with post-Lyme disease syndrome report a positive response to placebo. Furthermore, certain antibiotics, including doxycycline and ceftriaxone, used for treatment of this syndrome, have known anti-inflammatory effects unrelated to their antimicrobial properties, which may help alleviate some of the nonspecific symptoms. Some patients may simply feel subjectively better in time for other, unspecified reasons. Therefore, it is important to establish clear evidence of prior Lyme disease and distinguish from other factors that may be responsible for a patient's continued symptoms, including sleep disorders, depression, or symptoms attributable to other diagnosis, including fibromyalgia, chronic fatigue syndrome, or other spondyloarthropathies.[28,37]

Finally, treatment of post-Lyme disease syndrome is entirely supportive. A multidisciplinary approach can be very helpful to patients with symptoms of fatigue, myalgia, arthralgia, and cognitive manifestations. These treatments include emotional support, physical therapy, biofeedback, education on energy conservation techniques, implementation of an individualized graded exercise program, and other alternative therapies, including massage therapy and acupuncture.

SELF-ASSESSMENT

1. A 45-year-old man from Virginia presents in July with acute onset of drooling, which started 6 hours prior. One week ago, he experienced flulike symptoms, including a low-grade fever, headache, myalgia, arthralgia, and malaise. Those symptoms resolved after 4 days. He recalls going hiking with his wife before his illness, after which she found and removed an engorged tick from his buttocks 2 days later. His physical examination reveals left-sided facial nerve palsy. He has no rash. What is the most likely diagnosis?
   a. Early localized Lyme infection
   b. Early disseminated Lyme infection
   c. Late Lyme infection
   d. Herpes simplex virus reactivation

2. You decide to treat the above patient for B burgdorferi infection. Which of the following is the most suitable treatment regimen?
   a. Doxycycline for 14 days
   b. Doxycycline for 28 days
   c. Ceftriaxone for 28 days
   d. Erythromycin for 14 days

3. A 30-year-old forester from Wisconsin had a fever and erythema migrans in late June. He improved with 14 days of doxycycline. Now in September, he presents with fever and an erythematous patch on his buttocks. Serology is positive for Lyme disease. Which of the following is the most appropriate treatment at this time?
   a. Ceftriaxone for 14 days for a relapse
   b. Doxycycline for 6 weeks for a relapse
   c. Azithromycin for 21 days for a relapse
   d. Doxycycline for 10 to 21 days for a new infection

4. A 29-year-old woman who is 10 weeks pregnant returns from a week-long camping trip in Black Rock State Park, Connecticut. She now presents with fever, malaise, and an erythema migrans rash on her back. She has no drug allergies. What is the best course of treatment?
   a. Doxycycline for 14 days
   b. Amoxicillin for 14 days
   c. Ceftriaxone for 14 days
   d. No antibiotics
5. A 24-year-old woman from Boston has had extreme fatigue for the past 12 months. In addition, she has had chronic diffuse joint and muscle pain, sore throat, headaches, and palpitations. Her symptoms initially began in January and have persisted since. She was previously evaluated by her primary care physician, a rheumatologist, an ear, nose, and throat specialist, a neurologist, and a cardiologist with normal studies. She has been treated with several different antibiotic courses without improvement. Before her symptoms, she was an active marathon runner and a doctoral candidate in chemistry. Her physical examination is normal. A prior Lyme serology obtained at the onset of symptoms and again 3 months into her illness was positive for IgM antibodies and remains negative for IgG antibodies to *B burgdorferi*. What is the most likely diagnosis?
   a. Chronic fatigue syndrome
   b. Early disseminated Lyme disease
   c. Late Lyme infection
   d. Depression

Answers
   Answer 1: *B.*
      This patient is presenting with facial nervy palsy, a known neurologic manifestation of Lyme disease. Although he likely acquired early localized infection 1 week prior, he has progressed to the early disseminated form in the absence of treatment. The time course is too early for late Lyme infection. Herpes simplex virus reactivation can be a cause of cranial nerve palsy; however, the patient's presentation and exposure history suggest Lyme disease.
   Answer 2: *A.*
      Treatment of early Lyme infection is doxycycline for 14 days. In patients with more severe disseminated disease, such as significant AV nodal block, or meningitis, ceftriaxone for 28 days would be the agent of choice to start with. Erythromycin is an option for patients who have a contraindication to doxycycline, which this patient is not known to have.
   Answer 3: *D.*
      Most people who live in Lyme disease–endemic areas are at risk for re-exposure. There has been concern that Lyme disease can relapse, and that such relapses may require a prolonged course of therapy to eradicate the residual focus of infection. However, studies of patients who have experienced more than one episode of documented Lyme disease have shown that repeated episodes are in fact due to reinfections rather than a relapse. This episode should therefore be treated like the initial episode with doxycycline for 10 to 21 days. Amoxicillin or cefuroxime are alternatives in the case of allergy.
   Answer 4: *B.*
      This woman has early localized infection with Lyme disease. Doxycycline is a pregnancy category D drug, demonstrating teratogenicity in animal studies, and should be avoided in pregnant women. The alternatives would be

amoxicillin or cefuroxime (both category B). IV ceftriaxone is not indicated for early localized Lyme disease.

Answer 5: *A.*

Chronic fatigue syndrome or fibromyalgia needs to be considered for individuals with debilitating fatigue and multisystem organ symptoms after evaluation by multiple specialists without objective evidence of disease. Early disseminated Lyme disease would present with objective evidence of infection (inflammatory arthritis on examination if joint pain is present, AV nodal conduction abnormalities for cardiac involvement, and a positive serology confirmed by Western blot). Late Lyme infection would also demonstrate a positive serology, especially by 3 months of symptom onset. A life-altering medical event may lead to depression; however, depression in this case is considered secondary to the disability and not the primary problem.

REFERENCES

1. C.f.D.C.a.P. Reported cases of Lyme disease by year, United States, 1995–2013. 2015. Available at: http://www.cdc.gov/lyme/stats/chartstables/casesbyyear. html. Accessed September 16, 2015.
2. Steere AC, Sikand VK, Schoen RT, et al. Asymptomatic infection with Borrelia burgdorferi. Clin Infect Dis 2003;37(4):528–32.
3. Steere AC. Lyme disease (Lyme Borreliosis) due to Borrelia burgdorferi. In: Dolin R, Bennett JE, Blaser MJ, editors. Mandell, Douglas, and Bennett's principles and practice of infectious diseases. Philadelphia: Elsevier Saunders; 2015. p. 2725–35.
4. Nadelman RB, Nowakowski J, Forseter G, et al. The clinical spectrum of early Lyme borreliosis in patients with culture-confirmed erythema migrans. Am J Med 1996;100(5):502–8.
5. Strle F, Nadelman RB, Cimperman J, et al. Comparison of culture-confirmed erythema migrans caused by Borrelia burgdorferi sensu stricto in New York State and by Borrelia afzelii in Slovenia. Ann Intern Med 1999;130(1):32–6.
6. Steere AC, Sikand VK. The presenting manifestations of Lyme disease and the outcomes of treatment. N Engl J Med 2003;348(24):2472–4.
7. Shapiro ED. Lyme disease. N Engl J Med 2014;371(7):684.
8. Pachner AR, Steere AC. The triad of neurologic manifestations of Lyme disease: meningitis, cranial neuritis, and radiculoneuritis. Neurology 1985;35(1):47–53.
9. Halperin JJ. Nervous system lyme disease. Clin Lab Med 2015, in press.
10. Peeters N, van der Kolk BY, Thijsen SF, et al. Lyme disease associated with sudden sensorineural hearing loss: case report and literature review. Otol Neurotol 2013;34(5):832–7.
11. Fish AE, Pride YB, Pinto DS. Lyme carditis. Infect Dis Clin North Am 2008;22(2): 275–88, vi.
12. Steere AC, Schoen RT, Taylor E. The clinical evolution of Lyme arthritis. Ann Intern Med 1987;107(5):725–31.
13. Steere AC, Klitz W, Drouin EE, et al. Antibiotic-refractory Lyme arthritis is associated with HLA-DR molecules that bind a Borrelia burgdorferi peptide. J Exp Med 2006;203(4):961–71.
14. Stanek G, Strle F. Lyme borreliosis. Lancet 2003;362(9396):1639–47.
15. Asbrink E, Hovmark A, Olsson I. Clinical manifestations of acrodermatitis chronica atrophicans in 50 Swedish patients. Zentralbl Bakteriol Mikrobiol Hyg A 1986; 263(1–2):253–61.

16. Feder HM Jr, Johnson BJ, O'Connell S, et al. A critical appraisal of "chronic Lyme disease". N Engl J Med 2007;357(14):1422–30.

17. Klempner MS, Hu LT, Evans J, et al. Two controlled trials of antibiotic treatment in patients with persistent symptoms and a history of Lyme disease. N Engl J Med 2001;345(2):85–92.

18. Krupp LB, Hyman LG, Grimson R, et al. Study and treatment of post Lyme disease (STOP-LD): a randomized double masked clinical trial. Neurology 2003; 60(12):1923–30.

19. Kaplan RF, Trevino RP, Johnson GM, et al. Cognitive function in post-treatment Lyme disease: do additional antibiotics help? Neurology 2003;60(12):1916–22.

20. MacDonald AB. Human fetal borreliosis, toxemia of pregnancy, and fetal death. Zentralbl Bakteriol Mikrobiol Hyg A 1986;263(1–2):189–200.

21. Markowitz LE, Steere AC, Benach JL, et al. Lyme disease during pregnancy. JAMA 1986;255(24):3394–6.

22. Schlesinger PA, Duray PH, Burke BA, et al. Maternal-fetal transmission of the Lyme disease spirochete, Borrelia burgdorferi. Ann Intern Med 1985;103(1): 67–8.

23. Maraspin V, Cimperman J, Lotric-Furlan S, et al. Erythema migrans in pregnancy. Wien Klin Wochenschr 1999;111(22–23):933–40.

24. Lakos A, Solymosi N. Maternal Lyme borreliosis and pregnancy outcome. Int J Infect Dis 2010;14(6):e494–8.

25. Nadelman RB, Hanincová K, Mukherjee P, et al. Differentiation of reinfection from relapse in recurrent Lyme disease. N Engl J Med 2012;367(20):1883–90.

26. Wormser GP, Masters E, Nowakowski J, et al. Prospective clinical evaluation of patients from Missouri and New York with erythema migrans-like skin lesions. Clin Infect Dis 2005;41(7):958–65.

27. Morgan M, Nathwani D. Facial palsy and infection: the unfolding story. Clin Infect Dis 1992;14(1):263–71.

28. Wormser GP, Dattwyler RJ, Shapiro ED, et al. The clinical assessment, treatment, and prevention of lyme disease, human granulocytic anaplasmosis, and babesiosis: clinical practice guidelines by the Infectious Diseases Society of America. Clin Infect Dis 2006;43(9):1089–134.

29. Dever LL, Jorgensen JH, Barbour AG. In vitro antimicrobial susceptibility testing of Borrelia burgdorferi: a microdilution MIC method and time-kill studies. J Clin Microbiol 1992;30(10):2692–7.

30. Wormser GP, Ramanathan R, Nowakowski J, et al. Duration of antibiotic therapy for early Lyme disease. A randomized, double-blind, placebo-controlled trial. Ann Intern Med 2003;138(9):697–704.

31. Dattwyler RJ, Luft BJ, Kunkel MJ, et al. Ceftriaxone compared with doxycycline for the treatment of acute disseminated Lyme disease. N Engl J Med 1997; 337(5):289–94.

32. Karlsson M, Hammers-Berggren S, Lindquist L, et al. Comparison of intravenous penicillin G and oral doxycycline for treatment of Lyme neuroborreliosis. Neurology 1994;44(7):1203–7.

33. Ljostad U, Skogvoll E, Eikeland R, et al. Oral doxycycline versus intravenous ceftriaxone for European Lyme neuroborreliosis: a multicentre, non-inferiority, double-blind, randomised trial. Lancet Neurol 2008;7(8):690–5.

34. Donta ST. Macrolide therapy of chronic Lyme disease. Med Sci Monit 2003;9(11): PI136–42.

35. Donta ST. Tetracycline therapy for chronic Lyme disease. Clin Infect Dis 1997; 25(Suppl 1):S52–6.

36. Fallon BA, Tager F, Fein L, et al. Repeated antibiotic treatment in chronic Lyme disease. J Spirochetal Tick-Borne Dis 1999;5:94–102.
37. Girschick HJ, Guilherme L, Inman RD, et al. Bacterial triggers and auto-immune rheumatic diseases. Clin Exp Rheumatol 2008;26(1 Suppl 48): S12–7.

Nervous System Lyme Disease

John J. Halperin, MD[a,b],*

KEYWORDS

- Nervous system • Lyme disease • Neuroborreliosis
- Garin Bujadoux Bannwarth syndrome • Spinal fluid • Diagnosis • Treatment

KEY POINTS

- Lyme disease affects the nervous system in 10% to 15% of infected patients.
- Neuroborreliosis is qualitatively similar in patients infected with US and European strains.
- After the first 3 to 6 weeks of infection, peripheral blood 2-tier serologic testing (enzyme-linked immunosorbent assay with positives/borderlines confirmed by Western blot) is highly sensitive and specific.
- Measurement of intrathecal antibody production (ratio of the proportion of cerebrospinal fluid to serum specific anti–*Borrelia burgdorferi* antibody) is highly specific. Sensitivity is not established but is probably high in central nervous system inflammatory disease.
- Treatment with oral doxycycline is probably effective in most cases of neuroborreliosis.

BACKGROUND

What we do not understand frightens us. For many patients, the most dreaded, difficult-to-comprehend medical disorders are those that affect the nervous system; losing our cognitive abilities or our self-sufficiency is often more frightening than dealing with cancer or heart disease.[1] Unfortunately, many non-neurologist physicians also find neurology intimidating and inexplicable, presumably because of its complexity and quite likely because of the way it is taught in medical school. When patients present with difficult-to-explain symptoms, and their physicians struggle to understand the underlying pathophysiology, there is a tendency to leap to the assumption that the disorder is neurologic. This phenomenon is particularly common with disorders affecting behavior, in which patient symptoms may be out of proportion to objective clinical findings. These symptoms that can arise for medical, physiologic,

The author has nothing to disclose.
[a] Department of Neurosciences, Overlook Medical Center, 99 Beauvoir Avenue, Summit, NJ 07902, USA; [b] Sidney Kimmel Medical College of Thomas Jefferson University, 132 South, 10th street, Philadelphia, PA 19107, USA
* Department of Neurosciences, Overlook Medical Center, 99 Beauvoir Avenue, Summit, NJ 07902.
E-mail address: john.halperin@atlantichealth.org

Clin Lab Med 35 (2015) 779–795
http://dx.doi.org/10.1016/j.cll.2015.07.002
0272-2712/15/$ – see front matter © 2015 Elsevier Inc. All rights reserved.

labmed.theclinics.com

psychological, or other reasons.[2] What the physician often does not appreciate, however, is that by suggesting that the disorder is neurologic, patients' anxiety levels increase substantially, confounding, if not amplifying, the symptoms.

Much the same can be said of Lyme disease, perhaps because so much is made of what is thought to be nervous system involvement. Because of the focus of attention on the protean nature of Lyme disease, on how it is the great imitator, and how it can cause a subtle encephalopathy, these considerations have come to dominate the conversation.[3,4] This circumstance has led to a remarkably confrontational atmosphere between patient advocacy groups and mainstream medicine—a confrontation that embodies the tensions between evidence-based and anecdote-based medicine and between patient advocacy and engagement in medical decision making versus fact-based diagnosis and treatment. This infusion of fear of neurologic disease into the conversation about what in the 1970s was a new and poorly understood infectious disease has fueled a debate that shows little sign of abating.

Donald Rumsfeld famously referred to 'known knowns, known unknowns and unknown unknowns.'[5] The one permutation he omitted is the one that can best address the concerns associated with Lyme neuroborreliosis: the unknown knowns. In fact, there is a large body of information that should be informing this debate. Unfortunately, however, it is misunderstood or completely unknown to many involved in these discussions.

NEUROLOGY 101

Many disorders affect nervous system function; most are not neurologic. Neurologic disease encompasses the broad range of disorders that affect the structure, macroscopic or microscopic, of the peripheral or central nervous systems (PNS or CNS, respectively). Because of the limited regenerative capacity of the nervous system, these disorders tend to cause losses of function that either have limited reversibility or are progressive. In contrast to these intrinsic disorders of the nervous system, disordered nervous system function is ubiquitous. We have all experienced slowed cognition and impaired memory with fatigue, stress, and medical illness. All clinicians appreciate that patients with prominent immune activation, such as those with high fever and a significant infection, be it pneumonia, sepsis, or pyelonephritis, can be confused and exhibit surprisingly impaired function, impairment that disappears with resolution of the infection. Similarly, psychiatric disease can impact an individual's behavior and ability to function. Although many psychiatric disorders may fundamentally be neurochemical, at least at this time these are considered non-neurological disorders, as there is no demonstrable neuroanatomic substrate and because treatment and natural history of psychiatric and neurologic disorders are so fundamentally different.

Differentiating among neurologic disease, psychiatric disorders and the behavioral concomitants of systemic (non-neurologic) disease are usually straightforward.[2] The confusional state of medical illness is typically fairly acute in onset, fluctuates in time, and includes impairment of memory and orientation but does not seem to affect specific structures or localized functions of the brain. The behavioral abnormalities of psychiatric disease rarely affect orientation, at the extreme can include hallucinations and other evidence of disordered thought processes, but, again, do not affect specific structures or localized functions of the brain. Neurologic disease affects structures or systems; for example, a stroke or tumor can affect speech, unilateral strength, vision, or coordination, depending on location of the insult. A neuropathy affects strength, sensation, and reflexes in a pattern that follows neuroanatomic logic. Amyotrophic lateral sclerosis, Parkinson, and Alzheimer disease each affect specific functionally linked structures in the nervous system. The patient-perceived deficits in neurologic disorders can almost always be confirmed by a good clinical neurologic examination, which can be supplemented with appropriately selected laboratory and neurophysiologic testing (eg, electromyography or nerve conduction tests for PNS disease and neuroimaging for many focal CNS disorders). It is a basic tenet of clinical neurology that neurologic disorders can be confirmed by objective clinical means. Superimposed medical illnesses can be addressed by combining the neurologic conclusions with an appropriate medical evaluation. Psychiatric disorders can be more complex to diagnose precisely but can generally be differentiated from neurologic ones without much difficulty.

LYME DISEASE AFFECTING THE NERVOUS SYSTEM OR NEUROBORRELIOSIS

Patients infected with *Borrelia burgdorferi*, or the closely related European strains *B afzelii* and *B garinii* and the recently identified *B bavariensis*, can experience altered nervous system function by one of 2 mechanisms.[6] First are disorders caused by direct involvement of the CNS or PNS, in which there may be focal neurologic abnormalities alone or in combination with meningeal inflammation (meningitis). Such disorders must be differentiated from difficulties with memory, mental focus, and complex cognition that can occur with any significant, non-nervous system infection. The term *Lyme encephalopathy* was coined specifically to differentiate the latter disorder from brain infection or encephalitis.[7,8] This encephalopathy is not unique to or diagnostic of Lyme disease and should not be considered a manifestation of neuroborreliosis, a term that should be reserved specifically for nervous system infection with *B burgdorferi* or the other aforementioned species. Although there are numerous anecdotal reports of psychiatric disorders occurring in patients with Lyme disease, there is no epidemiologic evidence that Lyme disease is more common in patients with psychiatric illness or data to support that any specific psychiatric diagnosis is more common in patients with Lyme disease.[9,10] Presumably Lyme disease, similar to other illnesses or stressors, may precipitate an episode of psychiatric illness. The mechanism by which this occurs is unclear, but there are no data to suggest a unique association between Lyme disease and any psychiatric diagnoses.

A third syndrome, referred to as *chronic Lyme disease* (CLD), has often been attributed to nervous system infection with *B burgdorferi* or other tick-borne pathogens.[11] The constellation of clinical symptoms to which this term has been applied, including fatigue, pain, and difficulty with memory, concentration, and cognition, among other symptoms, is real, often disabling, and not uncommon. Notably, these symptoms can overlap with those of Lyme encephalopathy. However, when the term *CLD* is used to describe patients without clinical, laboratory, or even epidemiologic support for the diagnosis of Lyme disease, or for patients who have been successfully treated for Lyme disease, there is little to suggest that these symptoms are caused by ongoing infection with *B burgdorferi* or any other identified tick-borne pathogen. Whether the symptomatically similar disorder referred to as posttreatment Lyme disease syndrome is real or not remains to be determined.[12]

HISTORIC BEGINNINGS
The First Described Case of Neuroborreliosis

In 1922, Garin and Bujadoux[13] described a 58-year-old French sheep farmer who, 3 weeks following a tick bite, developed a rapidly enlarging erythroderma that expanded to involve his buttocks (site of the bite), adjacent abdomen, and most of his left thigh.[13] The patient also experienced radicular pain involving the bilateral sciatic and intercostal nerves. He subsequently developed excruciating pain in the right shoulder and arm, which was unresponsive to morphine. These symptoms persisted unabated; when evaluated 2.5 months later, he had marked right deltoid weakness and atrophy. Reflexes and sensory examination were normal despite continued, severe neuropathic pain in the shoulder, low anterior rib cage, and sciatic nerve distribution. Analysis of the patient's cerebrospinal fluid (CSF) revealed pleocytosis (75 white cells with polymorphonuclear leukocyte predominance), mild elevation of protein (130 mg/dL), and a slightly positive Wasserman test (a nontreponemal assay for syphilis). After a lengthy discussion explaining why they considered syphilis excluded, the investigators concluded that the patient suffered from a nonsyphilitic spirochetal infection and treated him with neoarsphenamine, the arsenic-containing compound used as standard management of neurosyphilis at the time. The excruciating pain resolved immediately following the first neoarsphenamine injection. Although the investigators confused this entity with tick-bite paralysis and added a parenthetic remark suggesting that spirochetes were viruses, this remains one of the best clinical descriptions of neuroborreliosis. Subsequent case series emphasized the involvement of cranial nerves as well, particularly the facial nerve.[14] Collectively, this triad of meningitis, radiculoneuritis, and cranial neuritis, described in more detail later (see Clinical manifestations), encompasses the most common manifestations of neuroborreliosis.

Lyme Pathophysiology

Although it is helpful to approach neuroborreliosis syndromically (ie, dividing presentations into those involving the PNS vs the CNS then by clinical presentation within those constructs), it is informative to start from a more general pathophysiologic perspective. Nervous system infections are generally uncommon, primarily because of the protective mechanisms provided by both anatomic (eg, skull, spine, and so forth) and cellular/intercellular barriers. The latter, consisting of the blood-brain and blood-nerve barriers, exclude most infectious organisms from gaining entry into the CNS, although some agents take advantage of a few chinks in the armor. The blood-nerve barrier is somewhat less complete than the blood-brain one, with gaps in the dorsal root ganglia and at the motor endplates. Polio, for example, takes advantage of these deficiencies, binding to motor nerve terminals to be transported proximally; herpes viruses invade sensory neurons and survive indefinitely in the dorsal root ganglia.

One of the challenges in understanding the pathophysiology of B burgdorferi nervous system infection has been the difficulty to consistently isolate viable organisms from either patients or experimentally infected rhesus macaque monkeys, which, to date, is the only experimental model of nervous system infection with B burgdorferi.[15–17] Even in patients with pronounced Lyme meningitis, organisms are detected in CSF by either culture or polymerase chain reaction (PCR) methods in only 10% to 15% of cases.[15,18,19] Detailed studies using histologic-, immunocytochemical-, culture-, and PCR-based techniques have had tremendous difficulty in identifying these spirochetes in involved peripheral nerves, the meninges, or CNS parenchyma.[17] Yet, active infection is clearly an essential element in the pathophysiology of neuroborreliosis, as appropriate antimicrobial therapy leads to rapid improvement in many objective measures of nervous system involvement, with ongoing amelioration of symptoms, if not complete resolution of deficits. Of course, as with any nervous system insult, deficits cannot be reversed until the damaged structure regenerates (in the PNS) or remyelinates, so immediate recovery should not be expected.

Histology of affected structures generally demonstrates multifocal and perivascular inflammation. There is rarely any blood vessel wall necrosis to allow a diagnosis of vasculitis. Neither spirochete antigens nor complement are typically demonstrable at the sites of inflammation.[20–22] This circumstance has resulted in several hypotheses regarding the pathophysiology of disease.

Several studies have found immunologic cross reactivity between various neuronal epitopes and *B burgdorferi sensu stricto* antigens, leading to suggestions of molecular mimicry, a mechanism thought to play a role in some patients with posttreatment Lyme arthritis.[23–25] However, the resolution of nervous system inflammation after antimicrobial treatment and the absence of a chronic inflammatory state analogous to post-treatment antibiotic-unresponsive arthritis would seem to make such a mechanism improbable. There is some evidence that *B burgdorferi* might bind to gangliosides and oligodendroglia, providing a potential mechanism for localization of the infection.[26,27] However, in the PNS, demyelinating neuropathies are at best rare, making it improbable that this mechanism underlies the observed broad range of PNS disorders. In the CNS, parenchymal involvement in cases of neuroborreliosis is likewise extremely rare, making it unlikely that *B burgdorferi* affinity for oligodendroglia is an important consideration.

On the other hand, the inflammatory response associated with neuroborreliosis often seems out of proportion to the number of demonstrable organisms. Studies suggest the following sequence of events. Through a mechanism that is to date not fully understood, *B burgdorferi* penetrates the blood-brain barrier easily and quite early in infection.[28] This penetration triggers local production of CXCL13, a B-cell–attracting chemokine, which then leads to early and substantial migration of B cells into the CNS where they multiply and develop into clones producing antibodies targeting *B burgdorferi*.[29–31] These clones persist in producing specific antibody long after the infection and related symptoms have resolved, with demonstrated persistence for up to a decade following curative treatment.[32] If clinical signs and symptoms were caused by these antibodies cross-reacting with neural structures, nervous system inflammation and disease might be expected to last as long as antibodies persist rather than resolving rapidly with administration of antibiotics (or even of arsenic).

Other studies suggest that either systemic or local production of various cytokines might play a pathophysiologic role, although specific mechanisms remain to be elucidated. Interferon γ and tumor necrosis factor α production may be increased during infection with potential downstream biochemical effects.[33] Some have suggested that patients with elevated interleukin 23 during infection may be more likely to have persistent symptoms after treatment.[34] Other work suggests that active infection results in elevated serum concentrations of CXCL9 and CXCL10.[35] The implications, or even the reproducibility, of these observations remain to be determined. However, it seems likely that immune activation plays an important role in amplifying the clinical impact of the small number of spirochetes that actually persist in the nervous system.

LABORATORY DIAGNOSIS OF NEUROBORRELIOSIS

The laboratory diagnosis of non-neuroinvasive Lyme disease is well described elsewhere in this issue.[36,37] Although laboratory confirmation of nervous system involvement is an imperfect science, there are helpful tools that can be applied in appropriate circumstances. The most common approach is to examine the CSF, as the associated findings are useful *if the CNS is infected*. It is critically important to realize, however, that in patients with primarily PNS involvement, including cranial neuritis, although the CNS may be involved, this is not invariable.[38] Hence, the finding of a completely normal CSF profile in a patient with peripheral nerve disease is informative as evidence that the CNS is uninvolved. However, this finding neither supports nor eliminates the possibility of PNS infection.

A

```
vvvvvvvvvvvvvvvvv  |  v
yyyyyyyyyyyyyyyyyyy  |  y
yyyyyyyyyyyyyyyyyyy  |  y
yyyyyyyyyyyyyyyyyyy  |  y
yyyyyyyyyyyyyyyyyyy  |  y
yyyyyyyyyyyyyyyyyyy  |  y
yyyyyyyyyyyyyyyyyyy  |  y
yyyyyyyyyyyyyyyyyyy  |  y
yyyyyyyyyyyyyyyyyyy  |  y
yyyyyyyyyyyyyyyyyyy  |  y
```

Blood   Brain

B

```
vvvvvvvvvvvvvvvvvv  |  v
yyyyyyyyyyyyyyyyyyyy  |  y
yyyyyyyyyyyyyyyyyyyy  |  y
yyyyyyyyyyyyyyyyyyyy  |  y
yyyyyyyyyyyyyyyyyyyy  |  y
yyyyyyyyyyyyyyyyyyyy  |  y
yyyyyyyyyyyyyyyyyyyy  |  y
yyyyyyyyyyyyyyyyyyyy  |  y
yyyyyyyyyyyyyyyyyyyy  |  y
yyyyyyyyyyyyyyyyyyyy  |  y
```

```
                                         B   B   B
                                         vvvvvvvvvvvvvv
                                         vvvvvvvvvvvvvv
```

Blood   Brain

C

```
vvvvvvvvvvvvvvvvv  |  vvv
yyyyyyyyyyyyyyyyyyyy  |  yyy
yyyyyyyyyyyyyyyyyyyy  |  yyy
yyyyyyyyyyyyyyyyyyyy  |  yyy
yyyyyyyyyyyyyyyyyyyy  |  yyy
yyyyyyyyyyyyyyyyyyyy  |  yyy
yyyyyyyyyyyyyyyyyyyy  |  yyy
yyyyyyyyyyyyyyyyyyyy  |  yyy
yyyyyyyyyyyyyyyyyyyy  |  yyy
yyyyyyyyyyyyyyyyyyyy  |  yyy
```

Blood   Brain

That said, in patients with Lyme meningitis or with parenchymal CNS involvement (ie, brain or spinal cord infection), CSF analysis can be informative in several ways. As with any active CNS infection, there should be a CSF pleocytosis, with lymphocyte predominance (though polymorphonuclear leukocytes may be present as in the case reported by Garin and Bujadoux[13]). Protein levels are usually modestly elevated (100–200 mg/dL), whereas glucose levels are typically normal to slightly low. Because of the predominant B-cell stimulation and the potentially protracted nature of the infection, it is not uncommon to see elevated overall production of immunoglobulin, resulting in an elevated immunoglobulin G (IgG) synthesis rate and even oligoclonal bands.[39] Notably, both of these findings are much more frequently described in patients infected with the European *Borrelia* strains.

The most specific test for Lyme neuroborreliosis is the assessment of specific anti–*B burgdorferi* antibody production within the CSF, referred to as the CSF:serum antibody index, a reflection of intrathecal antibody production (**Fig. 1**).[39–43] Because a small proportion (about 0.5%–1.0%) of peripheral blood IgG antibodies normally leaks into the CSF, simply measuring anti–*B burgdorferi* antibody in CSF is insufficient and inappropriate. Anti–*B burgdorferi* IgG antibodies will routinely be reported as positive in the CSF of patients with elevated serum antibodies or in whom blood-brain barrier leakage has occurred for other reasons—the 2 circumstances in which defining the role of *B burgdorferi* infection is most critical. Addressing this requires measuring the *proportion* of IgG antibodies specific to *B burgdorferi* in both CSF and serum. The intuitively simplest approach is to first dilute the CSF and serum to the same final total IgG concentration, then measure the specific anti–*B burgdorferi* antibody levels in both samples, followed by calculation of the CSF to serum antibody ratio. If the ratio is greater than 1.0, this indicates that specific anti–*B burgdorferi* antibodies are being produced in the CNS, whereas if the ratio is less than 1.0, the detected antibody is most likely present because of leakage into the CSF from blood. From a practical perspective, this can be done more simply with a capture enzyme immunoassay, a method that inherently measures the *proportion* of antibody specific to the target

◀——————————————————————————

Fig. 1. Intrathecal antibody production. (*A*) Normal: Blood-brain barrier allows 0.5% to 1.0% of IgG from blood to enter the CSF. Therefore, if 10% of blood antibody is specific to a given antigen, 10% of CSF antibody will be also. To compensate for these normal concentration differences, laboratories typically dilute serum 1:500 and CSF 1:1, so that postdilution IgG concentrations are, on average, identical. Subsequently, enzyme-linked immunosorbent assays (ELISAs) for antibodies specific to a given antigen will also have the same values in diluted serum and CSF (ie, CSF:serum ≤ 1.0). Note that because CSF values are compared with serum normal controls, in patients with elevated serum antibodies, CSF antibodies will be similarly elevated and interpreted as positive compared with normal; but CSF:serum ≤ 1.0 (not elevated). (*B*) Intrathecal antibody production: If a particular antigen enters the CSF, it will be followed by B cells producing targeted antibodies. The CSF concentration of this antibody will now equal the amount of antibody passively entering into the CSF as described in part (*A*) plus the locally produced antibody (ie, the concentration will exceed the amount entering passively). Thus, the CSF:serum ratio for the target antibody will be greater than 1.0. (*C*) Nonspecifically inflamed meninges allow more IgG to cross the blood-brain barrier. If the laboratory does not correct for this, the usual dilution of CSF 1:1 will leave a much higher concentration of IgG in the diluted CSF. If, for example, leakage allows the CSF IgG concentration to triple, then customary 1:1 dilution will result in the postdilution CSF IgG concentration being 3 times the expected value and ELISA results for any antibody will increase correspondingly, giving many false positives. (*Courtesy of* John J. Halperin MD, Summit, NJ; with permission.)

antigens.[43] Regardless of the technique used, it is essential to measure both CSF and serum antibodies, adjusting for blood-brain barrier permeability.

The neuroborreliosis antibody index method is quite specific. False positives may occur in cases of neurosyphilis; however, measuring reaginic antibodies (rapid plasma reagin, VDRL) will differentiate between these two spirochetoses. In theory other spirochetal infections can similarly cause cross-reactions, though fortunately there is little epidemiologically overlap.

There are 2 major shortcomings of the neuroborreliosis antibody index technique. First, measurable intrathecal production of specific antibody can continue for a decade after successful treatment.[32] Therefore, as with peripheral blood serology, a positive result cannot be used to differentiate between current and past infection. Fortunately active infection almost always elicits a CSF pleocytosis, so this provides a useful measure of disease activity. The second and perhaps more significant challenge is that in the absence of another gold standard diagnostic test, the sensitivity of the antibody index technique cannot be determined. In Europe, demonstration of intrathecal antibody production is a requirement for the diagnosis of definite neuroborreliosis.[44] As a result, sensitivity is by definition 100%. In a US study of Lyme meningitis, sensitivity of the assay was found to be approximately 90%,[45] whereas another study evaluating its utility in a broader spectrum of disorders reported a sensitivity of approximately 50%.[46] For now the actual sensitivity is indeterminate and remains an important area in need of clarification.

CLINICAL MANIFESTATIONS

Although it has become commonplace to refer to Lyme disease as the great imitator with protean manifestations, this reflects an approach to neurologic diagnosis based on symptom cataloging rather than pathophysiologic understanding.[47] Evaluation of potential cases of neuroborreliosis should begin with a consideration of whether infection involves the PNS versus CNS, recognizing that in a given patient either or both may be affected.

Peripheral Nervous System Involvement

Involvement of cranial or peripheral nerves occurs in approximately 10% of infected but untreated individuals and typically manifests quite early in infection.[48] In experimentally infected rhesus macaque monkeys, virtually all animals develop at least transient PNS disease.[49] Histopathology of affected peripheral nerves in experimental monkeys, and in the few human biopsies that are available, demonstrates patchy perineural and perivascular lymphocytic infiltrates.[21,22] Although a few small series provide neurophysiologic evidence of Guillain-Barre–like demyelination, all experimental and virtually all clinical data demonstrate a multifocal inflammatory disorder with loss of axons, a mononeuropathy multiplex (**Table 1**).[38,50,51] Clinical presentations include the following:

Radiculitis

As originally described by Garin and Bujadoux,[13] and subsequently by Bannwarth,[14] 3% to 5% of patients will present with acute neuropathic-type pain, typically radicular in character and localization.[52] The European literature suggests that Garin Bujadoux Bannwarth syndrome commonly involves the dermatome associated with the site of the tick bite (corresponding data are not available for the United States). As in the original description, pain can be intractable and the dominant symptom, but muscle denervation and reflex loss can also occur. Typically findings involve one or a few adjacent dermatomes. When severe, the corresponding spinal cord level can also become involved, causing myelopathic symptoms and findings.

Table 1	
PNS manifestations of neuroborreliosis	
Clinical Manifestation	**Pathophysiology**
Cranial neuritis (VII, V, III, IV, VI, VIII) Radiculitis (1 or several contiguous dermatomes) Plexopathy (brachial, lumbosacral) Mononeuritis Mononeuritis multiplex Stocking glove (confluent mononeuropathy multiplex)	Mononeuritis multiplex (multifocal inflammation)
Demyelinating neuropathy	Association rare and questionable

Cranial neuritis

Cranial neuropathies, particularly involving (facial) nerve VII, occur slightly more frequently. Lyme disease, along with Guillain-Barre syndrome, sarcoidosis, and basilar meningitides, is one of the few causes of bilateral facial nerve palsies, which can occur simultaneously or in close temporal sequence. Less commonly, the cranial nerves to the extraocular muscles can be involved, causing diplopia, the trigeminal nerve may be affected, causing numbness or pain in the face, or the vestibulo-acoustic nerve can be damaged, leading to imbalance. Notably, the optic nerve is rarely if ever affected; lower cranial nerve involvement is limited to isolated case reports only.[53–55]

Mononeuropathy

Some patients develop a typical mononeuropathy or mononeuropathy multiplex: focal involvement of one or several individual peripheral nerves. Occasionally, this can involve the brachial or lumbosacral plexus, the complex structures in which the nerves to the limbs form from the originating spinal nerve roots.

Confluent mononeuropathy multiplex

European patients with acrodermatitis chronica atrophicans, a disorder not described in the United States, can develop a multifocal peripheral neuropathy, typically presenting with widespread, yet somewhat asymmetric sensory symptoms that slowly evolve into a stocking glove–type presentation[50] with symptoms gradually ascending from the fingers and toes, to the hands and feet, then more proximally. This disorder is histologically and physiologically identical to the stocking glove–type neuropathy described in US patients with long-standing Lyme disease. In both cases, it is probably a variant of a mononeuropathy multiplex in which many small nerves are involved, known as a confluent mononeuropathy multiplex.

Detailed neurophysiologic studies in a large cohort of patients with all forms of PNS Lyme involvement indicate that all have a mononeuropathy multiplex, including patients with cranial neuropathies and radiculitis, varying only in severity and anatomic distribution.[38]

Central Nervous System Involvement

As described in the earliest cases, lymphocytic meningitis following *B burgdorferi* invasion of the CNS is quite common and can occur either in isolation or together with PNS manifestations (**Table 2**). Symptoms of this meningitis are quite variable and bear little relation to CSF cell count; some patients with modest pleocytosis can have severe headaches, photophobia, and neck stiffness, and others with a more pronounced pleocytosis may be entirely asymptomatic. Presumably symptoms are more related to cytokine release in the CSF, though further studies are needed to elucidate this.

Table 2
CNS manifestations of neuroborreliosis

Clinical Manifestation	Pathophysiology
Meningitis	Meningeal seeding with *B burgdorferi*
Pseudotumorlike (children primarily)	Meningitis with increased intracranial pressure
Myelitis	Multifocal inflammatory extension from involved nerve root
Parenchymal brain involvement (very rare)	Multifocal inflammation

For children in particular, meningitis caused by *B burgdorferi* infection can be accompanied with raised intracranial pressure and present with a picture resembling pseudotumor cerebri.[56–58] Patients develop papilledema and headaches and can have visual obscurations or visual loss. CSF evaluation in most demonstrates a pleocytosis. Because the term *pseudotumor cerebri* refers to a noninflammatory elevation in intracranial pressure, this *B burgdorferi*–related disorder might be better referred to as pseudo-pseudotumor. Management must address the intracranial pressure as well as the infection.

Rarely, patients may develop parenchymal brain or spinal cord inflammation. Described primarily in the 1970s and 1980s,[42,59,60] before the advent of reliable diagnostic tools and treatment, this manifestation most commonly involved the spinal cord segments contiguous to afflicted nerve roots in patients with Garin Bujadoux Bannwarth syndrome. Rarely cerebral, cerebellar or brain stem involvement was also evident. Generally, localization was clinically evident and confirmed by MRI, which demonstrated focal areas of active inflammation.[42,59,60] In the 1980s and 1990s, the incidence of such inflammation was estimated at 1 case per million population at risk per year. With widespread early treatment, the incidence of cerebral involvement today appears to be even less.

Lyme Encephalopathy

In the 1980s, when it was commonplace to see patients with longstanding Lyme arthritis, it was noted that many with this ongoing inflammatory state described difficulties with cognition, memory, and overall intellectual function. Many were exhaustively evaluated for possible CNS involvement; for virtually all patients' clinical examinations, CSF findings, and imaging studies were completely normal.[7,8,46] Given the similarity of this state to the toxic-metabolic encephalopathy seen in patients with other inflammatory states (ranging from lupus to bacterial pneumonia) and given the absence of any evidence of CNS infection in affected individuals, the disorder was termed *Lyme encephalopathy*.[7,42,61] It was studied extensively in the hope that this might shed light on the pathophysiology of other inflammation-associated encephalopathies.

Unfortunately this construct was widely misunderstood. Labeling the clinical entity Lyme encephalopathy led some to assume that the pattern of cognitive difficulty is specific to Lyme disease or, even worse, diagnostic of it. Describing it in the context of CNS Lyme disease, even though the data showed that affected individuals *did not have CNS infection*, compounded the misunderstanding. Although neither of these assumptions was ever a consideration in the original descriptions, it has become commonplace in some circles to assume that these symptoms alone are sufficient to diagnose CNS Lyme disease and to treat accordingly. This notion has been expanded further such that individuals without any epidemiologic possibility of exposure to *B burgdorferi* and no laboratory evidence of infection are treated for an extended period of time for a disease they do not have. Sadly, when they fail to respond, they receive ever more complex and potentially toxic regimens.

Posttreatment Lyme Disease Syndrome and Chronic Lyme Disease

An outgrowth of this misinterpretation of the implications of Lyme encephalopathy has been the creation of 2 diagnostic labels: posttreatment Lyme disease syndrome (PTLDS) and CLD.[12,62] It was recognized early on that in many patients who were appropriately and successfully treated for Lyme disease, nonspecific symptoms could take weeks to months to resolve (not unlike patients with other significant infections). The suggestion that, in some individuals, symptoms might persist for 6 months or longer led to the creation of the rubric PTLDS, defined as "the presence of any of: widespread musculoskeletal pain, cognitive complaints, radicular pain, paresthesias, or dysesthesias. . . interfering with. . . function. . . within 6 months after. . . initial diagnosis and treatment. . . and. . . persisting for at least 6 months."[12] Notably, however, these symptoms have been found to be at most *minimally* more frequent in patients treated for Lyme disease as compared with a control population, whereas all objective findings were identical in patients and controls.[63–65] A recent study in patients with well-defined and treated Lyme disease found this disorder to be extremely rare.[66] Most importantly, it has been clearly demonstrated that additional treatment for Lyme disease does not provide a meaningful benefit for these patients.[67–69]

The label CLD, although not precisely defined, has been applied to individuals with symptoms similar to PTLDS but who typically lack any basis for a diagnosis of Lyme disease. The greatest challenge here is that these symptoms, which overlap entirely with those of chronic fatigue syndrome or, to use the nomenclature recently recommended by the Institute of Medicine, systemic exertion intolerance disease,[70] are highly prevalent in the general population. Studies indicate that at any given time approximately 2% of the population has these symptoms to a degree that is significantly disabling.[70,71] Labeling these patients as suffering from a variant of Lyme disease has been a relief to many, as it provided a biological label for their disabling disorder and a potential treatment plan. However, beyond the lack of evidence that their symptoms are attributable to *B burgdorferi* infection, the added incorrect notion that these symptoms are a result of nervous system infection substantially elevates their fears, creating the belief they have a very difficult-to-treat neurodegenerative disorder. Repeated statements that Lyme disease can mimic anything, including Lou Gehrig disease, multiple sclerosis, and Alzheimer disease, build on this fear and paradoxically serve to elevate patients' confidence in the practitioners they come to view as the brave few who have finally diagnosed them correctly and offered treatment. The fact that these practitioners' opinions are rejected by the broad medical community only serves to reinforce the sense that modern medicine has failed these highly symptomatic patients. Even when treatment fails, these patients retain hope of cure when they are told that this is a notoriously difficult-to-treat infection, requiring additional complex regimens. When they suffer adverse events caused by treatment, such as a drug fever, this is explained as a Herxheimer reaction, which is the acute inflammatory reaction seen in some infections when many infectious organisms are suddenly killed by effective antimicrobial therapy, which is considered confirmatory evidence of their response to treatment.

As more and more evidence accumulates to indicate that chronic Lyme disease cannot be attributed to chronic *B burgdorferi* infection, some practitioners have turned to attributing them to infection with other tick-borne agents, including *Babesia* species, *Ehrlichia* species, *Anaplasma phagocytophilum*, and even some non–tick-borne organisms, including *Bartonella henselae*.[72] Neither the fact that these patients lack compelling clinical or laboratory evidence of infection with these agents nor the absence of evidence that these organisms cause chronic infections dissuades such practitioners from prescribing potentially toxic medications targeting these infections. Perhaps most paradoxically, the International Lyme and Associated Diseases Society's guidelines argue for aggressive, early treatment of erythema migrans with doxycycline, amoxicillin, or cefuroxime axetil, stating that successful treatment with any of these agents will prevent what they consider to be late manifestations of these coinfections.[62] Yet 2 of these 3 agents (amoxicillin and cefuroxime axetil) have no efficacy whatsoever against these pathogens.

TREATMENT OF LYME NEUROBORRELIOSIS

Treatment of Lyme disease has been addressed in Chapter 2 of this volume. One element that remains incompletely resolved, however, is whether oral antimicrobials are sufficient to treat nervous system disease. The need to treat CNS infection was the reason for the initial introduction of ceftriaxone for severe Lyme disease and remains the argument used for prolonged parenteral treatment by CLD-treating practitioners.[73] However, there are now multiple European studies indicating that, for Lyme meningitis, cranial neuritis, and radiculoneuritis, oral doxycycline, similar to parenteral ceftriaxone, is curative in approximately 95% of patients.[74] Although this has not yet been systematically evaluated in North American populations, the similarity between the infectious organisms and the known pharmacokinetics of doxycycline make it highly likely that oral doxycycline will likewise be effective in all but the most severe cases of neuroborreliosis.

SUMMARY

Lyme disease affects the PNS and CNS in 10% to 15% of European and US patients infected with *B burgdorferi*, *B afzelii*, and *B garinii*. Pathophysiologically, this consists of either lymphocytic meningitis or a multifocal inflammatory process. The latter affects the PNS frequently and the CNS quite rarely. In children, meningitis can result in elevated intracranial pressure, causing a pseudotumorlike picture. Diagnosis of CNS disease is best confirmed by CSF examination, whereby intrathecal production of anti–*B burgdorferi* antibodies is frequently demonstrable. Treatment, with either oral doxycycline or parenteral regimens, is highly effective.

SELF-ASSESSMENT

1. The most common clinical presentation of CNS infection with *B burgdorferi* is
   a. Encephalitis
   b. Encephalopathy
   c. Brachial plexopathy
   d. Meningitis
2. Which of the following is the least common manifestation of PNS neuroborreliosis:
   a. Demyelinating polyneuropathy
   b. Brachial plexopathy
   c. Mononeuropathy multiplex
   d. Painful radiculitis
3. Two-tier serologic testing (enzyme-linked immunosorbent assay [ELISA] with confirmatory Western blot) is least sensitive in

a. Erythema migrans
b. Lyme meningitis
c. Lyme cranial neuritis
d. Acrodermatitis related neuropathy
4. Measurement of intrathecal antibody production is best performed by
   a. Performing a standard ELISA (same method as serum) for antibodies to *B burgdorferi* on undiluted CSF and comparing the value to normal serum values
   b. As in (a) but comparing it to patients' serum ELISA
   c. Performing a Western blot on undiluted CSF and standard dilution serum
   d. Diluting serum so it has the same final IgG concentration as the patients' CSF and performing standard ELISAs for *B burgdorferi* antibodies on both
5. Treatment of nervous system Lyme disease
   a. Should always be with parenteral antibiotics
   b. Is often successful with oral doxycycline
   c. Is often successful with oral azithromycin
   d. Requires intravenous ceftriaxone

Answers
   Answer 1: d
   Answer 2: a
   Answer 3: a
   Answer 4: d
   Answer 5: b

REFERENCES

1. Marist.Poll. Alzheimer's most feared disease. 2012. Available at: http://maristpoll.marist.edu/1114-alzheimers-most-feared-disease/. Accessed August 31, 2013.
2. Halperin JJ. Lyme disease – neurology, neurobiology and behavior. Clin Infect Dis 2014;58(9):1267–72.
3. Pachner AR. Neurologic manifestations of Lyme disease, the new "great imitator". Rev Infect Dis 1989;6:S1482–6.
4. Logigian EL, Kaplan RF, Steere AC. Successful treatment of Lyme encephalopathy with intravenous ceftriaxone. J Infect Dis 1999;180(2):377–83.
5. Washington, DC: U.S. Department of Defense, Office of the Assistant Secretary of Defense (Public Affairs); 2002.
6. Margos G, Wilske B, Sing A, et al. Borrelia bavariensis sp. nov. is widely distributed in Europe and Asia. Int J Syst Evol Microbiol 2013;63(Pt 11):4284–8.
7. Halperin JJ, Krupp LB, Golightly MG, et al. Lyme borreliosis-associated encephalopathy. Neurology 1990;40:1340–3.
8. Krupp LB, Masur D, Schwartz J, et al. Cognitive functioning in late Lyme borreliosis. Arch Neurol 1991;48:1125–9.
9. Nadelman RB, Herman E, Wormser GP. Screening for Lyme disease in hospitalized psychiatric patients: prospective serosurvey in an endemic area. Mt Sinai J Med 1997;64(6):409–12.
10. Hassett AL, Radvanski DC, Buyske S, et al. Psychiatric comorbidity and other psychological factors in patients with "chronic Lyme disease". Am J Med 2009;122:843–50.
11. Lantos PM. Chronic Lyme disease: the controversies and the science. Expert Rev Anti Infect Ther 2011;9(7):787–97.

12. Wormser GP, Dattwyler RJ, Shapiro ED, et al. The clinical assessment, treatment, and prevention of Lyme disease, human granulocytic anaplasmosis, and babesiosis: clinical practice guidelines by the Infectious Diseases Society of America. Clin Infect Dis 2006;43:1089–134.

13. Garin C, Bujadoux A. Paralysie par les tiques. J Med Lyon 1922;71:765–7.

14. Bannwarth A. Chronische lymphocytare meningitis, entzundliche polyneuritis und "rheumatismus". Arch Psychiatr Nervenkr 1941;113:284–376.

15. Karlsson M, Hovind HK, Svenungsson B, et al. Cultivation and characterization of spirochetes from cerebrospinal fluid of patients with Lyme borreliosis. J Clin Microbiol 1990;28(3):473–9.

16. Avery RA, Frank G, Eppes SC. Diagnostic utility of *Borrelia burgdorferi* cerebrospinal fluid polymerase chain reaction in children with Lyme meningitis. Pediatr Infect Dis J 2005;24(8):705–8.

17. Roberts ED, Bohm RP Jr, Lowrie RC Jr, et al. Pathogenesis of Lyme neuroborreliosis in the rhesus monkey: the early disseminated and chronic phases of disease in the peripheral nervous system. J Infect Dis 1998;178(3):722–32.

18. Ogrinc K, Lotric-Furlan S, Maraspin V, et al. Suspected early Lyme neuroborreliosis in patients with erythema migrans. Clin Infect Dis 2013;57(4):501–9.

19. Cerar T, Ogrinc K, Cimperman J, et al. Validation of cultivation and PCR methods for diagnosis of Lyme neuroborreliosis. J Clin Microbiol 2008;46(10):3375–9.

20. Meier C, Grahmann F, Engelhardt A, et al. Peripheral nerve disorders in Lyme-Borreliosis. Nerve biopsy studies from eight cases. Acta Neuropathol (Berl) 1989;79(3):271–8.

21. Vallat JM, Hugon J, Lubeau M, et al. Tick-bite meningoradiculoneuritis: clinical, electrophysiologic, and histologic findings in 10 cases. Neurology 1987;37(5):749–53.

22. Halperin JJ, Little BW, Coyle PK, et al. Lyme disease - a treatable cause of peripheral neuropathy. Neurology 1987;37:1700–6.

23. Aberer E, Brunner C, Suchanek G, et al. Molecular mimicry and Lyme borreliosis: a shared antigenic determinant between Borrelia burgdorferi and human tissue. Ann Neurol 1989;26(6):732–7.

24. Sigal LH. Molecular mimicry and Lyme borreliosis [letter]. Ann Neurol 1990;28(2):195–6.

25. Martin R, Gran B, Zhao Y, et al. Molecular mimicry and antigen-specific T cell responses in multiple sclerosis and chronic CNS Lyme disease. J Autoimmun 2001;16(3):187–92.

26. Garcia-Monco JC, Seidman RJ, Benach JL. Experimental immunization with *Borrelia burgdorferi* induces development of antibodies to gangliosides. Infect Immun 1995;63(10):4130–7.

27. Garcia Monco JC, Wheeler CM, Benach JL, et al. Reactivity of neuroborreliosis patients (Lyme disease) to cardiolipin and gangliosides. J Neurol Sci 1993;117(1–2):206–14.

28. Luft BJ, Steinman CR, Neimark HC, et al. Invasion of the central nervous system by Borrelia burgdorferi in acute disseminated infection. JAMA 1992;267(10):1364–7.

29. Ljostad U, Mygland A. CSF B–lymphocyte chemoattractant (CXCL13) in the early diagnosis of acute Lyme neuroborreliosis. J Neurol 2008;255(5):732–7.

30. Rupprecht TA, Plate A, Adam M, et al. The chemokine CXCL13 is a key regulator of B cell recruitment to the cerebrospinal fluid in acute Lyme neuroborreliosis. J Neuroinflammation 2009;6:42.

31. Halperin JJ, Pacheco-Quinto J, Herdt A, et al. [S37.007] serum and CSF cytokines in patients with active CNS Lyme disease, other inflammatory CNS diseases, encephalopathy following treated Lyme disease, other encephalopathies, and normal controls. Am Acad Neurol 2015. Washington, DC.

32. Hammers Berggren S, Hansen K, Lebech AM, et al. *Borrelia burgdorferi*-specific intrathecal antibody production in neuroborreliosis: a follow-up study. Neurology 1993;43(1):169–75.

33. Halperin JJ, Heyes MP. Neuroactive kynurenines in Lyme borreliosis. Neurology 1992;42(1):43–50.

34. Strle K, Stupica D, Drouin EE, et al. Elevated levels of IL-23 in a subset of patients with post-Lyme disease symptoms following erythema migrans. Clin Infect Dis 2014;58(3):372–80.

35. Soloski MJ, Crowder LA, Lahey LJ, et al. Serum inflammatory mediators as markers of human Lyme disease activity. PLoS One 2014;9(4):e93243.

36. Schriefer ME. Lyme Disease Diagnosis: Serology. Clin Lab Med 2015, in press.

37. Alby K, Capraro GA. Alternatives to Serologic Testing for Diagnosis of Lyme Disease. Clin Lab Med 2015, in press.

38. Halperin JJ, Luft BJ, Volkman DJ, et al. Lyme neuroborreliosis - peripheral nervous system manifestations. Brain 1990;113:1207–21.

39. Henriksson A, Link H, Cruz M, et al. Immunoglobulin abnormalities in cerebrospinal fluid and blood over the course of lymphocytic meningoradiculitis (Bannwarth's syndrome). Ann Neurol 1986;20:337–45.

40. Stiernstedt GT, Granstrom M, Hederstedt B, et al. Diagnosis of spirochetal meningitis by enzyme linked immunosorbent assay and indirect immunofluorescence assay in serum and cerebrospinal fluid. J Clin Microbiol 1985;21: 819–25.

41. Hansen K, Lebech A-M. Intrathecal synthesis of Borrelia burgdorferi specific immunoglobulin G, A and M in neuroborreliosis - an antibody capture assay. Paper presented at: IV International Conference on Lyme Borreliosis 1990. Stockholm, Sweden, June 18–21, 1990.

42. Halperin JJ, Luft BJ, Anand AK, et al. Lyme neuroborreliosis: central nervous system manifestations. Neurology 1989;39(6):753–9.

43. Steere AC, Berardi VP, Weeks KE, et al. Evaluation of the intrathecal antibody response to Borrelia burgdorferi as a diagnostic test for Lyme neuroborreliosis. J Infect Dis 1990;161(6):1203–9.

44. Mygland A, Ljostad U, Fingerle V, et al. EFNS guidelines on the diagnosis and management of European Lyme neuroborreliosis. Eur J Neurol 2010;17(1): 8–16. e11–14.

45. Halperin JJ, Volkman DJ, Wu P. Central nervous system abnormalities in Lyme neuroborreliosis. Neurology 1991;41:1571–82.

46. Logigian EL, Kaplan RF, Steere AC. Chronic neurologic manifestations of Lyme disease. N Engl J Med 1990;323(21):1438–44.

47. Sanders L. Think like a doctor: mirror, mirror solved. New York Times 2014;2014.

48. Bacon RM, Kugeler KJ, Mead PS. Surveillance for Lyme disease — United States, 1992–2006. MMWR Morb Mortal Wkly Rep 2008;57(SS10):1–9.

49. England JD, Bohm RP, Roberts ED, et al. Mononeuropathy multiplex in rhesus monkeys with chronic Lyme disease. Ann Neurol 1997;41(3):375–84.

50. Hopf HC. Peripheral neuropathy in acrodermatitis chronica atrophicans (Herxheimer). J Neurol Neurosurg Psychiatry 1975;38(5):452–8.

51. Logigian EL, Steere AC. Clinical and electrophysiologic findings in chronic neuropathy of Lyme disease. Neurology 1992;42(2):303–11.

52. Krishnamurthy KB, Liu GT, Logigian EL. Acute Lyme neuropathy presenting with polyradicular pain, abdominal protrusion, and cranial neuropathy. Muscle Nerve 1993;16(11):1261–4.
53. Sibony P, Halperin J, Coyle P, et al. Reactive Lyme serology in patients with optic neuritis and papilledema. J Neuro Ophthal 2005;25(2):71–82.
54. Blanc F, Ballonzoli L, Marcel C, et al. Lyme optic neuritis. J Neurol Sci 2010;295: 117–9.
55. Djukic M, Larsen J, Lingor P, et al. Unilateral phrenic nerve lesion in Lyme neuroborreliosis. BMC Pulm Med 2013;13:4.
56. Nord JA, Karter D. Lyme disease complicated with pseudotumor cerebri. Clin Infect Dis 2003;37(2):e25–6.
57. Zemel L. Lyme disease and pseudotumor. Mayo Clin Proc 2000;75(3):315.
58. Jacobson DM, Frens DB. Pseudotumor cerebri syndrome associated with Lyme disease. Am J Ophthalmol 1989;107(1):81–2.
59. Ackermann R, Rehse KB, Gollmer E, et al. Chronic neurologic manifestations of erythema migrans borreliosis. Ann N Y Acad Sci 1988;539:16–23.
60. Ackermann R, Gollmer E, Rehse KB. Progressive Borrelia encephalomyelitis. Chronic manifestation of erythema chronicum migrans disease of the nervous system. Dtsch Med Wochenschr 1985;110(26):1039–42.
61. Halperin JJ, Pass HL, Anand AK, et al. Nervous system abnormalities in Lyme disease. Ann N Y Acad Sci 1988;539:24–34.
62. Cameron DJ, Johnson LB, Maloney EL. Evidence assessments and guideline recommendations in Lyme disease: the clinical management of known tick bites, erythema migrans rashes and persistent disease. Expert Rev Anti Infect Ther 2014;12(9):1103–35.
63. Seltzer EG, Gerber MA, Cartter ML, et al. Long-term outcomes of persons with Lyme disease. JAMA 2000;283(5):609–16.
64. Skogman BH, Croner S, Odkvist L. Acute facial palsy in children–a 2-year follow-up study with focus on Lyme neuroborreliosis. Int J Pediatr Otorhinolaryngol 2003;67(6):597–602.
65. Shadick NA, Phillips CB, Sangha O, et al. Musculoskeletal and neurologic outcomes in patients with previously treated Lyme disease. Ann Intern Med 1999; 131(12):919–26.
66. Wormser GP, Weitzner E, McKenna D, et al. Long-term assessment of fatigue in patients with culture-confirmed Lyme Disease. Am J Med 2015;128(2):181–4.
67. Klempner MS, Hu LT, Evans J, et al. Two controlled trials of antibiotic treatment in patients with persistent symptoms and a history of Lyme disease. N Engl J Med 2001;345(2):85–92.
68. Krupp LB, Hyman LG, Grimson R, et al. Study and treatment of post Lyme disease (STOP-LD): a randomized double masked clinical trial. Neurology 2003; 60(12):1923–30.
69. Fallon BA, Keilp JG, Corbera KM, et al. A randomized, placebo-controlled trial of repeated IV antibiotic therapy for Lyme encephalopathy. Neurology 2008;70: 992–1003.
70. Committee on the Diagnostic Criteria for Myalgic Encephalomyelitis/Chronic Fatigue Syndrome. Beyond myalgic encephalomyelitis/chronic fatigue syndrome: redefining an illness. Washington, DC: The National Academies Press; 2015.
71. Luo N, Johnson J, Shaw J, et al. Self-reported health status of the general adult U.S. population as assessed by the EQ-5D and Health Utilities Index. Med Care 2005;43(11):1078–86.

72. Telford SR 3rd, Wormser GP. Bartonella spp. transmission by ticks not established. Emerg Infect Dis 2010;16(3):379-84.
73. Dattwyler RJ, Halperin JJ, Volkman DJ, et al. Treatment of late Lyme disease. Lancet 1988;1:1191-3.
74. Halperin JJ, Shapiro ED, Logigian EL, et al. Practice parameter: treatment of nervous system Lyme disease. Neurology 2007;69(1):91-102.

Lyme Disease Diagnosis
Serology

Martin E. Schriefer, PhD

KEYWORDS

- Lyme disease • *Borrelia burgdorferi* • Serologic testing • Standard 2-tier testing
- Pitfalls • Predictive value serology

KEY POINTS

- Serology has been the mainstay of laboratory confirmation of Lyme borreliosis because direct detection of *Borrelia burgdorferi* has limited application.
- Although standardized 2-tier testing (STTT) detection of early, localized infection is poor, that of late disease is very good.
- The best indicator of stage 1 infection, erythema migrans, is presented in the majority of US cases; when recognized in a relevant epidemiologic setting, it should prompt treatment without testing.
- Clinical and epidemiologic correlates of infection should be carefully assessed before ordering STTT and for evaluation of its results.
- Efforts to simplify serologic testing include use of recombinant antigens and alternatives to STTT; these developments promise to improve performance, particularly in early disease detection.

INTRODUCTION

In 1982, the spirochetal agent of Lyme disease, later named *Borrelia burgdorferi*, was identified in and cultured from *Ixodes scapularis* ticks.[1] Shortly thereafter, it was cultured from blood, erythema migrans (EM) skin rash biopsies, and the cerebrospinal fluid of patients with differing stages of Lyme borreliosis in the United States and Europe using a modified media that had been developed in 1971 for propagation of relapsing fever spirochetes.[2–4] Although culture isolation from patients and animal model infection studies solidified the etiology of Lyme disease, this gold standard diagnostic has not proven to be a particularly sensitive approach for laboratory confirmation of infection in the United States.[5–7] This shortcoming for Lyme disease, although not uncommon in the field of bacterial etiologic agent recovery from clinical samples, is owing to the vanishingly small number of cultivable spirochetes in any

Bacterial Disease Branch, Division of Vector-Borne Disease, Centers for Disease Control and Prevention, 3156 Rampart Road, Fort Collins, CO 80521, USA
E-mail address: mms7@CDC.GOV

Clin Lab Med 35 (2015) 797–814
http://dx.doi.org/10.1016/j.cll.2015.08.001
0272-2712/15/$ – see front matter Published by Elsevier Inc.
labmed.theclinics.com

human tissue or fluid (often on the order <1/mL of blood in early disease) and that these numbers most often diminish with duration and dissemination of infection.[6] Differences in spirochete loads, persistence, and cultivability between vector ticks (certain *Ixodes* spp.), reservoir animals (such as *Peromyscus leucopus*) and dead-end hosts (such as *Homo sapiens*) are notable and prompt intriguing questions regarding the biology and survival mechanisms of this spirochete in its varied environments and possible approaches to better understand and improve human diagnostics and minimize disease.

With the varied tissues and organs potentially involved in human disease and the limitations of culture for laboratory confirmation of infection, alternative methods of diagnosis have been explored since the early 1980s. These include microscopy, immunohistochemistry, nucleic acid amplification, and immune response detection. This article provides an overview of the state of the diagnostic art for Lyme borreliosis, namely, serology, for the past 30 years. Most serology-specific understanding presented will focus on findings in North American patients infected with *B burgdorferi* sensu stricto (ss). Finally, recent advances and likely future directions for Lyme disease serodiagnostics are presented.

INFECTION AND IMMUNE RESPONSE

Natural Lyme borreliosis infection of humans and other mammals occurs over a period of hours and is initiated 1 to several days after the infected tick attaches to the host's skin and starts imbibing its blood. At this point in tick feeding, spirochetes residing in its midgut lumen are stimulated to replicate and migrate through the circulatory hemolymph to the salivary glands and finally into the skin of the host. Changes in spirochete gene expression and antigen profile occur during this migration as the spirochete prepares for its drastically altered environments and the defensive assault, both passive and active, awaiting in the mammalian host.[8,9] Through these physical, physiologic, and defensive processes, it is estimated that spirochetes from as few as 5% of infected ticks feeding on humans are transmitted successfully.[10] When successful, hundreds to thousands of bacteria may be inoculated over a multi-hour period before the tick terminates feeding. The likelihood of a continued infection and dissemination from the tick bite site is further reduced by both innate and active immunity. Despite these odds, without early and appropriate treatment, roughly 60% of *B burgdorferi*–infected patients in the United States will manifest disseminated infections with multiple EMs and other noncutaneous systems involvement (available: http://www.cdc.gov/lyme/signs_symptoms/index.html).

After infected tick feeding, the first indication of transmission and early infection in most North American patients is the development of an EM rash at the site of the previous tick bite. A rash developing within the first hours of tick attachment is not an EM or indicative of infection. EM development is a product of the innate immune response and occurs between 3 and 30 days after infection with an average of 7 days. The innate immune system is preprimed to recognize and quickly respond to a limited number of foreign patterns including those displayed by the outer surface proteins (Osp) of *B burgdorferi*.[11] Spirochete numbers (inoculated dose and subsequent replication) as well as their migration from the bite site factor into this early immune response and the subsequent EM appearance and behavior. Prospective and carefully attended patient studies indicate that EM occurs in about 85% or more of newly infected US Lyme patients, but is in practice less frequently observed and reported in nonstudy patients.[12,13] Reasons for discrepancies in EM detection include location (hidden or not frequently viewed anatomic sites), atypical or unrecognized appearance, and its transient nature. Multiple EMs, resulting from spirochete dissemination to skin sites distal to the prior tick bite, occur in less than 25% of North American patients.[12] Causes of other, EM-like, rashes include cellulitis in response to inoculation of skin flora or other microorganisms during the tick feeding, reactions to tick salivary proteins and a variety of skin reactions unrelated to tick bites.[14,15]

The adaptive immune response, leading in part to antibody production, is initiated within the first days of infection. However, antibody production in response to active infection is most often below the limits of current laboratory detection methods for at least 7 days. Thus, testing for antibody to B burgdorferi while the tick is still attached or several days thereafter is too early and will almost never yield a result with useful predictive (positive or negative) value. In addition to dependence on the duration of infection, measurable antibody responses are positively correlated with markers of spirochete dissemination and replication. Patients with multiple EMs and/or extracutaneous infections have more robust antibody titers and profiles than those with localized cutaneous infections.[16]

Most B burgdorferi antigens are protein or lipoprotein. The earliest detectable antibody responses are against OspC, flagellin B, and variable membrane proteinlike E (VlsE).[7] These, as most foreign proteins, display multiple antigenic determinants (epitopes), which elicit distinct antibody responses. Individual epitopes may be linear (5–6 amino acids) or conformational (disparate amino acid sequences brought into close proximity by protein folding) and unique to the protein or organism, or conserved among other proteins from the same or differing organisms. Proteins serving similar functions in differing organisms often have conserved features and antigenic determinants. The level of epitope uniqueness and its immunogenicity largely define its utility as a serodiagnostic marker of infection. B burgdorferi–specific linear epitopes may be identified by amino acid sequencing and then cloned away from the rest of the whole protein to produce peptide-based seroassays.[17,18] However, peptide cloning removes any conformational epitopes displayed by the larger, native protein. Thus, recombinant peptide-based seroassays must balance increased specificity with potentially lost conformational sensitivity.

During natural tickborne infection, most B burgdorferi antigens elicit an immunoglobulin (Ig)M and IgG response. IgM is the first antibody class produced in response to infection and the presence of IgG antibody alone is not suggestive of early infection. IgM is a pentavalent antibody (in contrast with bivalent IgG) and tends to produce higher background and crossreactivity than IgG in enzyme immunoassays (EIAs) and Western immunoblots. After several weeks of infection, IgG antibody displays increases in both quantitative (titer against specific antigens) and qualitative (number of reactive antigen) reactivity compared with IgM. During this time frame (several weeks to several months) both IgM and IgG are expected. IgG antibodies are characteristically of higher epitope affinity than their IgM predecessors.

SEROLOGY BEFORE 1995

Propagation of B burgdorferi in vitro requires specialized media and laboratory conditions. Soon after their recovery from patients, rodents, and ticks in the early 1980s, cultures were shared between clinical, field, and pharmaceutical investigators. These served as the starting materials of most commonly used assays developed to detect antibody responses to infection; whole-cell immunofluorescent assay, whole-cell sonicate (WCS) EIA, and Western immunoblot. As the field of Lyme disease diagnostics was developing and there was not yet general awareness of the effects of varied in vitro growth environments, passage, and storage on spirochete gene expression and stability, or the range of genetic diversity within the disease causing species, little attention was paid to the pedigree, history, and stability of culture isolates. Compounding the heterogeneous background of antigen starting materials was the parallel heterogeneity of Lyme disease patient's samples used to set test cutoffs and assess test performance. Although culture isolation was the gold standard for some early disease patient identifications, this was not a universal practice and recovery from later stages of disease was poor. Further, serodiagnostic result ambiguity arose around the common use of samples from patients that were collected months to years after antibiotic treatment and clinical cure. As has been since documented, antibody profiles persist in correlation with duration and dissemination of infection. Thus, although treated and cured, early disease patients are likely to have antibody profiles that diminished over the course of weeks to months, similarly treated and cured later disease patients typically maintain a robust antibody profile for months to years.

Using samples from patients with subjective Lyme disease histories or pooling of samples from true patients also led to errant conclusions regarding antibody evolution. Whereas the former diminished the specificity of tests in development, the latter compromised their ability to discern stage-specific immunity. For example, although patients with late Lyme arthritis almost always have strong antibody to OspA, early patients almost never do. Thus, whereas a test for Lyme arthritis may consider assessment of antibody to OspA, a test for early disease would waste resources and predictive value by measuring antibody to this antigen.

If characterization and inclusion criteria for positive controls were not challenging enough, those of negative controls were often ignored, oversimplified (eg, saline), or did not fully reflect a test-needy population (eg, only healthy individuals). Lyme disease epidemiology in this timeframe indicated that the human infections were rare and risk was geographically very limited. While the constellation of objective and subjective signs of infection was being more fully defined, it was underappreciated that the latter alone would soon describe some populations of patients with alternate etiologies that would seriously challenge the specificity of all laboratory testing for Lyme disease.

Many features of early Lyme disease serology tests (antigen or strain source, cutoffs, positive and negative controls, expected and separate IgM and IgG responses) were not standardized. This made comparative test performance very difficult. In 1990, the American Association of State and Territorial Public Health Laboratory Directors (ASTPHLD), the Centers for Disease Control and Prevention (CDC) and, the US Food and Drug Administration (FDA) cosponsored the First National Conference on Lyme Disease Testing in Dearborn, Michigan.[19] This meeting brought together more than 120 US research scientists, manufacturers, and representatives from state and federal agencies to address the problems associated with Lyme disease testing. Four recommendations were made: (1) develop a reference collection of samples from culture-confirmed and clinically characterized Lyme disease patients, obtaining serial samples when practical, (2) develop improved methods for isolating B burgdorferi from clinical material, (3) convene a conference on the use of serologic test methods, and (4) convene a working group to standardize serologic test methods.[19]

The need to meet these recommendations was underscored in a publication reporting on proficiency testing performance from hospitals, independent laboratories, physician offices, and manufacturers.[20] At this time point, there were more than a dozen major pharmaceutical suppliers of Lyme disease tests, from whom more than 30 assays had received FDA clearance between 1987 and 1992. The variety of available assay formats and analytes was challenging to select from and included whole-cell immunofluorescent assays, WCS-EIAs, purified protein (eg, p39) EIAs, and Western immunoblots, as well as choices for measuring IgM, IgG. or IgM and IgG antibodies. With the lack of standardization and the number of possible test choices, it was of little surprise that wildly varying performance was reported. In 1 study, Lyme disease samples were missed by close to 55% of the tests used and up to 27% of the healthy subject samples yielded false-positive results in certain tests.[20] In 1993, the CDC convened a Work Group on Standardization of Serodiagnosis of Lyme disease, which included participants from 5 academic laboratories offering Lyme disease serology. Over the next year, each of the participants tested 600 blind-coded samples from Lyme disease patients and controls by EIAs and Western immunoblots (findings presented elsewhere in this article).[21]

By the early 1990s, at least a dozen studies reporting Western immunoblot antibody reactivity in US Lyme disease patients had been published.[22–26] This diagnostic approach sought to capitalize on the resolving power of polyacrylamide gel electrophoresis (PAGE) and the ability to measure antibody against the resolved proteins in transfer (Western) immunoblots. PAGE was capable of resolving more than 50 B burgdorferi proteins, largely on the basis of their molecular weights, and more than 20 of them were found to react with antibodies from infected patients. Separate assessment of IgM and IgG antibody to each of the antigens was also easily afforded. However, no blotting criteria for positive identification of patients were yet established. Several studies in the early 1990s set benchmarks for both criteria and performance of Lyme disease diagnostic assays. In 1993, a study by Dressler and colleagues[25] analyzed separate IgM and IgG Western immunoblot reactivity to 14 of the most commonly reactive antigens of cultured B burgdorferi with samples from more than 200 Lyme disease patients (early localized and disseminated to late neurologic and arthritic disease) and controls (healthy and alternate [non-Lyme] disease). Based on blot data from these samples receiver operator characteristics curves, plotting sensitivity versus specificity, for antibody reactivity to distinct antigens was defined for Lyme disease patients and control groups. For early disease IgM Western immunoblots were most sensitive and specific by requiring reactivity to 2 or more of 8 specific antigens (bands), whereas for disease beyond several weeks of duration, IgG Western immunoblots meeting reactivity to 5 or more of 10 specific bands displayed the best discriminatory ability. This study also linked antibody profiles with disease stages and system (eg, cutaneous, neurologic, joint) involvement and highlighted the nonspecificity of antibody to some B burgdorferi antigens among patients with other diseases or healthy populations. Under the described criteria the IgM blot had a sensitivity of 32% and specificity of 100% in early disease, whereas the IgG blot had a sensitivity of 83% and specificity of 95% for later disease.[25] The study results underscored the ability of immunoblotting to shed light on samples with equivocal or false positive EIA results. A separate immunoblot study by Engstrom and colleagues,[26] focusing on serially collected serum samples from early disease EM patients, found optimal IgM Western immunoblot performance by requiring reactivity to at least 2 of 3 B burgdorferi proteins and that patient samples collected 8 to 12 days after diagnosis and the initiation of antibiotic treatment had the highest levels of reactive antibody. A parallel multicenter evaluation by the CDC Work Group found that the most accurate results were obtained by using an EIA supplemented by Western immunoblot.[21,27] Further, this study revealed that not all strains of B burgdorferi performed equally well as seroantigen sources. These studies and others culminated in the discussions and recommendations of the Second National Conference on Serologic Diagnosis of Lyme Disease in 1994 and the 1995 MMWR recommendations for test performance and interpretation.[28,29]

STANDARDIZED 2-TIER TESTING

The 1995 MMWR recommendations for Lyme disease test performance and interpretation formulated a standardized 2-tier testing (STTT) approach whereby serum samples were tested with a sensitive first-tier EIA or IFA followed by IgM and IgG Western immunoblot of first-tier positive or equivocal samples. It was further stipulated that IgM Western immunoblot use be restricted to patients with early disease and a duration of 30 days or less. IgM Western immunoblot positive criteria required reactivity to 2 or 3 of 3 antigens (p21 [OspC], p39 [BmpA] and p41 [flagellin B])[26] and IgG Western immunoblot criteria required reactivity to 5 or more of 10 antigens (p18, p21 [OspC], p28, p30, p 39 [BmpA], p41 [flagellin B], p45, p58, p66, and p93).[25] Under the 1994 Dearborn standardization recommendations, only *B burgdorferi* strains documented to produce ample amounts of each of the Western immunoblot criteria antigens were acceptable for immunoblot preparation. Provisions were also made for the acceptance of new tests that displayed equivalent or improved sensitivity, specificity, and precision to replace 1 or both components of the STTT.[28] Several resources collected by the CDC were made available to assist with test standardization and evaluation and included a panel of sera from well-documented Lyme disease patients and a set of monoclonal antibodies to *B burgdorferi* antigens for Western immunoblot calibration.

STANDARDIZED 2-TIER TESTING PERFORMANCE, 1995 TO PRESENT

Since implementation of the STTT for Lyme disease serology and interpretation in the United States, standardization and performance have improved.[30] Nonetheless, the disease presentation and testing can be complex. Several excellent reviews are available to assist physicians in the best use of available tests in the context of possible clinical settings.[31,32] Understanding the performance of reported serology is complicated by the variety of analytical tests used and the sample sets used to establish their performance, and the range of media reviews on the topic.

A summary of 2-tier performance as a function of disease stage is shown in **Table 1**. Data shown represent more than a dozen reviewed and primary studies published over a 20-year time frame between 1993 and 2013.[7,33–39] Lyme disease patients in the included studies were clinically and epidemiologically well-defined and in many cases the diagnosis *B burgdorferi* infection was independently confirmed by culture and/or polymerase chain reaction. IgM Western blot use was restricted to the first 30 days of illness.

It is readily apparent in **Table 1** that STTT sensitivity in early illness is poor. In this timeframe of disease onset and humoral immune response, a low rate of seropositivity is expected. It is also expected and observed that STTT sensitivity increases from

Table 1
Standardized 2-tier testing sensitivity and specificity

Early Disease (% Positive)			Late Disease (% Positive)	Controls (% Negative)
Stage 1[a]		Stage 2	Stage 3	Non-Lyme Disease
Acute EM	Convalescent EM			
17–40	27–78	40–100	96–100	98.0–100

Abbreviation: EM, erythema migrans.
  [a] Where stage 1 localized and disseminated infections were discriminated in the original publication a mean was calculated.
  Data from Refs.[7,33–38]

acute to convalescent stage 1 infection and further in stage 2 infection. What perhaps is not expected is the large range of sensitivity observed in stage 1 (17%–78%) and stage 2 (40%–100%) samples. Although this performance range has led some to question the accuracy and reproducibility of all tests for Lyme disease, several studies have revealed the spirochetal and host immune response causes behind it.[35,40,41] Early Lyme disease in the United States is most often (≥85%) manifested with EM. In addition, patients may have evidence of localized or disseminated infection.[40,41] Using the criteria of Massarotti, localized infection is defined as EM with no more than regional lymphadenopathy, fatigue, or minor headache, whereas disseminated infection is defined as secondary EM(s), arthritis or arthralgia, abdominal pain or tenderness, generalized lymphadenopathy, or signs of central nervous system involvement (headache and neck stiffness, facial palsy, or dysesthesias).[42] In published studies plotting STTT performance as a function of disease duration for both localized or disseminated infections, it is clear that organismal dissemination (and presumably replication) and duration of infection (days to weeks) are direct correlates of antibody response.[16,35]

A study by Wormser and colleagues[35] using acute, pretreatment sera from single or multiple EM patients assessed their rates of STTT positivity (**Table 2**). Patients were further delineated by duration of EM (1–4 weeks) before enrollment and culture confirmation. In patients with single EM of 1 week or less duration, STTT positivity was only 14%. This rate increased significantly in other single EM patients as a function of time before treatment, peaking at 86% for patients with 22 to 30 days of EM.[35]

For patients with disseminated disease, as assessed by multiple EMs in this study, with 1 week or less of duration, STTT was significantly higher at 65% compared with single EM patients at 14%.[35] Interestingly, the rate of STTT positivity did not increase among multiple EM patients with a longer duration of EM before treatment. These findings and those of similar studies suggest that, among patients with early disease, presenting to the physician with EM evidence of disseminated infection, the antibody response (as measured by STTT) has already peaked.[35,43] Unfortunately, in most studies these clinical correlates are not delineated or displayed and only the stage of illness is. By grouping all stage 1 disease serologies together, it is not possible to appreciate the impact of dissemination and duration of infection on the rate of seropositivity. However, as revealed in **Table 2**, these are important pretest assessments and the knowledgeable physician may use them to gauge the value of testing and testing results. For further discussion of pretesting and posttesting metrics see Predictive Value of Serology Results.

Stage 2 illness is defined by extracutaneous infection that may involve the neurologic, cardiac, or rheumatologic systems. The time from infection to manifested

Table 2
STTT sensitivity as function of single or multiple EM duration

EM Presentation	Duration of EM Before Testing and STTT Sensitivity (% Positive)			
	1–7 d	8–14 d	15–21 d	22–30 d
Single	14.1	33.3	33.3	85.7
Multiple	65.4	62.5	75.0	33.2

Abbreviations: EM, erythema migrans; STTT, standardized 2-tier testing.
Data from Wormser GP, Nowakowski J, Nadelman RB, et al. Impact of clinical variables on *Borrelia burgdorferi*-specific antibody seropositivity in acute-phase sera from patients in North America with culture-confirmed early Lyme disease. Clin Vaccine Immunol 2008;15(10):1520.

involvement of 1 or more of these systems may be as short as a couple weeks to as long as several months. As in stage 1 patients, the duration of infection is expected to impact seroreactivity in stage 2 patients; again, a large range of STTT positivity (40%–100%) is observed. The low end of STTT sensitivity is in part owing to the 30-day restricted use of IgM Western immunoblots.[29] Although the exact timing of illness onset is often difficult to pinpoint, several studies suggest a slightly extended (1–2 weeks) usefulness of IgM Western immunoblots.[33,44]

Not shown in **Table 1** or **2** are the individual sensitivities of IgM and IgG Western immunoblots in early disease. Again, these both are directly correlated to duration and dissemination of infection. However, the vast majority of positive STTT findings in early disease depend on positive IgM Western immunoblots; although most patients will develop IgG antibody detectable in Western immunoblots, only a minority will meet positive IgG Western immunoblot criteria at the time of clinical diagnosis.[16,35]

Stage 3 illness in the United States is most commonly presented as Lyme arthritis and much less so as late neuroborreliosis. STTT sensitivity in this stage of disease is very good (96%–100%) and specificity of properly applied and performed STTT is as well (98%–100%; see **Table 1**). As in the case of stage 2 illness, it is observed that for stage 3 infection the antibody response is very robust. Only rarely do well-documented stage 3 patients fail to meet STTT criteria. It must be recognized, however, that positive STTT results do not equate to persistent infection. The antibody profile in most stage 2 and 3 patients will persist for many months after effective treatment and cure.

PITFALLS IN STANDARDIZED 2-TIER TESTING

The complexity of STTT for Lyme borreliosis may result in its misuse and misunderstanding. Some of the more commonly observed pitfalls and errors in use and interpretation of STTT are presented in this section.

Testing Too Soon After Early Infection

Testing of individuals who have just removed a tick, even if the individual is infected, is highly unlikely to yield a serology result with a useful predictive value. A detectable antibody response takes at least several days to develop and studies have shown that less than 15% of patients with localized disease will have a positive STTT result within the first week of onset of illness. However, once initiated, the antibody response will continue to mount, even in the face of curative antibiotic treatment, over the course of several weeks. Several studies have demonstrated that patients treated early in the course of localized disease will display maximal titers of antibody 8 and 14 days later.[16,26,35]

Single-Tier Testing

A variety of first-tier tests have received FDA clearance. Historically, most first-tier test have been WCS EIAs. These tests may be fully or partially automated and are still in popular use. In general, they display high sensitivity but inadequate specificity. For greatest test result accuracy, the STTT should be used as well. Use of a first-tier test, or a second-tier test as a standalone will reduce specificity as compared with STTT.

Immunoglobulin M Western Immunoblotting Regardless of Duration of Illness

Many laboratories only perform first-tier testing for Lyme disease. Thus, first-tier reactive samples are often forwarded from first-tier sites to sites that offer Western immunoblot testing. Although recommendations advise against performing IgM Western immunoblots in cases with illness duration of greater than 30 days,[29] onset and sample collection information may not be conveyed or considered when Western immunoblots are performed. It is thus important for the physician to consider these recommendations and understand their basis when interpreting test data. Time-limited use of IgM Western immunoblots is owing to the less specific nature of this test compared with IgG Western immunoblots. Among healthy individuals with no risk of Lyme disease, IgM Western immunoblots generate a false-positive standalone test result about 5% of the time and higher rates of false positivity are seen among patients with alternate disease etiologies. Dependence on IgG Western immunoblot is based on the expectation that patients with greater than 30 days of untreated infection will have a robust IgG profile.

Overinterpretation of Less Than Positive Standardized 2-tier Testing Results

Another misguided practice is to assume that any reactivity short of a positive interpretation (most commonly in Western immunoblots) is still suggestive of B burgdorferi infection. Most, if not all, B burgdorferi antigens have epitopes that are conserved or crossreactive with antigens of other organisms. For example, low levels of IgG reactivity to p41 (flagellin B) are present in the serum of about 50% of tested healthy subjects. Caution and an alternate etiology should be considered when reviewing less than positive test reactivity.

POSTTREATMENT TESTING

Currently there are no validated seroassays for assessment of cure. Seroprofiles will slowly diminish after effective treatment. However, the time course of this process, although dependent on the duration and dissemination of infection before treatment, is not defined clearly. Further, in early stages of disease, it is common to see increases in humoral immunity over a period of several weeks after initiation of antibiotics because the immune process, once initiated, will continue to mount. In common with many infectious diseases, clinical resolution of signs may take months and this slow resolution should not be taken as an indicator of continued infection. In rare cases, retreatment may be necessary and further expansion of the humoral profile may support such a decision.

DEVELOPMENTS SINCE 1995 AND STANDARDIZED 2-TIER TESTING

Once established, B burgdorferi infection may to persist for months to years despite an active immune response. Although long-hypothesized, antigenic variation as a means to immune evasion and persistence was not documented for B burgdorferi until the discovery and characterization of an expressed variable major protein, VlsE.[45] This surface exposed lipoprotein, which is not expressed in useful amounts for EIA or Western immunoblot in in vitro cultures, is encoded by the 28-kb linear plasmid of B burgdorferi. VlsE contains variable and invariable antigen domains and within one of these variable domains there are 6 invariable regions (IR1–6). The IRs are conserved in the B burgdorferi sensu lato (sl) complex and the most conserved of these IRs, IR6, is immunodominant in infected humans and other mammals.[46] The whole VlsE protein or a 26-mer synthetic peptide (C6) within the IR6 sequence have been used extensively to assess antibody evidence of infection with B burgdorferi in the United States and elsewhere (**Table 3**).[7,36,39,43,46] The repeated findings of C6 sensitivity as good as or better than (particularly in early disease) 2-tier testing have been published. Similar performance between C6 and VlsE

Table 3
Comparative sensitivity and specificity of C6 and STTT

	Early Disease Sensitivity (% Positive)			Late Disease Sensitivity (% Positive)	Control Specificity (% Negative)
	Stage 1[a]		Stage 2	Stage 3	
	Acute EM	Convalescent EM	Neuritis or Carditis	LA or Late NB	
C6	29–74	56–90	60–100	94–100	97.2–100
STTT	17–40	27–78	40–100	96–100	98.0–100

Abbreviations: EM, erythema migrans; LA, lyme arthritis; NB, neuroborreliosis; STTT, standardized 2-tier testing.
[a] Where stage 1 localized and disseminated infections were discriminated in the original publication a mean was calculated.
Data from Refs.[7,33–38]

is also reported.[7,43] Although the specificity of C6 (or VlsE) assays is much greater than WCS-EIAs (data not shown), it is slightly less than that of STTT in some studies (see **Table 3**). In 2001, the C6 assay was approved as a first-tier test by the FDA and its use in place of WCS-EIA continues to increase.

At least 5 other first-tier assays, based on combinational use of purified or recombinant VlsE and OspC (or portions thereof), have been cleared by FDA since 2001. As with the C6 assay discussed, these approaches take advantage of the specificity and immunogenicity of these antigens and the ability to present them in differing formats away from the many less specific antigens of whole cell preparations. For listing of FDA 510(k) cleared tests for the detection of antibody to *B burgdorferi*, enter "LSR" in product code at the website http://www.accessdata.fda.gov/scripts/cdrh/cfdocs/cfPMN/pmn.cfm.

Western immunoblotting for Lyme disease is considered technically complex owing to the number of hands-on procedural steps required and the need to visually score final immunoblot reactivity for up to 10 bands. Efforts to minimize its complexity have used purified native or recombinant antigens in line blots as well automated scanning and scoring. By applying purified antigens to blotting supports one is able to avoid the physical overlap of some antigens common in PAGE Western immunoblots and deliver desired amounts of each antigen instead of accepting the variable amounts produced by cultured organisms. Also, by using densitometric scanning and software driven scoring, cutoffs for each antigen can be preprogrammed, taking the human reader out of the equation. FDA 510(k) cleared immunoblot assays for Lyme disease can be found by entering LSR in the product code at the website http://www.accessdata.fda.gov/scripts/cdrh/cfdocs/cfPMN/pmn.cfm.

Two-tier Enzyme Immunoassays

In view of the pitfalls and complexity of Western immunoblot, a 2011 study by Branda and colleagues[37] made a comparative analysis of STTT and a 2-EIA approach (WCS EIA followed by C6 EIA). Numerous published performance evaluations of the C6 assay had shown similar or better sensitivity, but slightly less specificity, compared with the STTT approach.[7,33,36,39] It was postulated that, by using a 2-EIA approach, one might maintain the specificity observed in STTT while improving on its sensitivity. This was in fact was what was found with greatest improvements in early (stage 1 and 2) disease detection. For stage 1 samples, the 2-EIA approach detected 63% as compared with 42% detection for STTT. Similarly, for stage 2 illness, the 2-EIA testing identified 100% of patients compared with only 40% detected by STTT. Both approaches displayed 100% detection of stage 3 Lyme disease (late Lyme arthritis and late Lyme neuritis) and 99.5% specificity (healthy and non-Lyme, disease controls). In addition to performance improvement for early disease, the 2-EIA approach offered a simple and quantitative result as compared with the technically complex features of Western immunoblots in the STTT approach and their semiquantitative output. Two-EIA performance was also presented as part of an independent study by Wormser and colleagues.[39,47] Very similar to the findings by Branda and colleagues, WCS EIA followed by C6 EIA detected 61% of stage 1 cases compared with 35% detection by STTT. Likewise, 90% of stage 2 samples were detected by 2-EIA compared with 80% by standard 2-tier testing. The findings of these 2 studies are summarized in **Table 4**. Together, assessing well over 4000 samples from Lyme disease patients, diseased and healthy controls, they offer strong support for the improved sensitivity performance of a 2-EIA approach over the STTT while maintaining the high specificity characteristic of the latter.

Centers for Disease Control and Prevention Lyme Serum Repository

In 2013, the CDC made available serum sets from a large (>400) and diverse population of well-characterized Lyme disease patients and control subjects for the purpose of test development and validation.[48] Samples from US patients representing all stages of Lyme disease were collected at diagnosis and before antibiotic treatment. Wherever possible, patient infections were confirmed by nonserologic methods including culture and/or polymerase chain reaction. Clinical presentations and histories were collected for all patients. In addition to Lyme disease patient samples, serum samples from patients with other diseases that may overlap clinically with Lyme disease or generate antibody responses that may crossreact in Lyme disease serodiagnostic assays were collected. Also included in the repository are samples from healthy persons residing in Lyme disease endemic and nonendemic areas of the country. All samples, Lyme patient and others, were tested by STTT and results of those serologies are available. Samples and supporting clinical and serologic data can be obtained together or samples can be obtained in a coded fashion for the purpose of blinded test performance evaluation.

Predictive Value of Serology Results

The predictive value of a test result (how often a positive or negative result is likely to be true) goes far beyond the sensitivity and specificity of the tests themselves in that it

Table 4
Comparative test sensitivity and specificity

Sample Type	No. Samples Tested	WCS EIA	C6	Standardized 2-tier Testing	2-EIA
Stage 1[a,b]	529	74.0 (73.0–74.9)	67 (66.5–67.5)	38.6 (35.2–42.0)	61.8 (60.5–63.0)
Stage 2[a]	30	97.5 (95–100)	95 (90–100)	60 (40–80)	95 (90–100)
Stage 3[a]	140	97.5 (95–100)	99.2 (98.4–100)	98 (95.9–100)	98.8 (97.5–100)
Controls[c]	3541	96.3 (95.3–97.3)	98.7 (98.4–98.9)	99.5 (99.5)	99.5 (99.5)

Mean (range) from Refs.[37,39,47] For reference[37] phase 1 study results are included.
Abbreviations: WCS EIA, whole-cell-sonicate enzyme immunoassay.
[a] Percent positive.
[b] Mean of acute and convalescent sensitivity.
[c] Percent negative.

is additionally dependent on the pretest probability. If a test has both 100% sensitivity and 100% specificity, pretest clinical and epidemiologic measures have no impact on the predictive value of results. Short of these extreme test performance metrics, and in situations of disease prevalence other than 100% or 0%, test result predictive value is variable and depends on the physician's pretest assessment of both clinical and epidemiologic correlates.[49–51]

Pretest probability ranges over logs of scale for both epidemiologic and clinical correlates. In the highest risk areas of the country, which are very rare, incidence may be on the order of several percent, whereas in regions of disease cycle absence, the incidence is zero. Between these extremes is the continuum of risk and incidence. US reported case maps are available online (at http://www.cdc.gov/lyme/stats/index.html). Similar to epidemiologic pretest probability is the continuum of clinical pretest probability, ranging from close to 100% to well below 0.001%. Objective clinical correlates of high value (eg, recurrent and brief attacks of swelling in 1 or a few joints, cranial nerve palsy, acute onset, high-grade heart conduction defects) in an epidemiologic risk environment will significantly increase the pretest likelihood of disease. Yet, even these results may be more often caused by something other than Lyme disease. By example, onset of facial palsy during summer months in Long Island, New York, a region of high epidemiologic risk, was found to have other, non-Lyme disease, causes in close to 75% of cases.[52] Other less specific correlates of Lyme disease (eg, arthralgia, myalgia, headache, fatigue, paresthesia, mildly stiff neck, heart palpitations, and myocarditis), particularly when presented alone, are of very minimal pretest probability value. Thus, for extracutaneous manifestations of Lyme disease in the context of significant epidemiologic risk, laboratory testing may greatly assist the physician's diagnosis. However, when presented with the same case in the context of low epidemiologic risk, the physician must be aware that positive test results are often misleading.[50]

Although a precise and accurate pretest likelihood assessment is difficult and may be argued among subject matter experts, a relative pretest probability need not be. **Fig. 1** portrays the predictive value positive and negative of 4 tests (WCS-EIA, C6, STTT, and 2-EIA) as a function of pretest probability for each stage of Lyme borreliosis. As reviewed in **Tables 1–3**, the sensitivity of serologic tests presented increases from stage 1 to stage 2 and stage 3. In parallel with increased test sensitivity, the predictive value positive for all tests increases. This stage-dependent increase is most apparent at low (<20%) pretest probabilities. It is further observed in this low pretest range (up to ~20%) that the predictive values positive increase sharply as the pretest probability increases. However, the impact of epidemiologic risk must be kept in mind; positive results in similar cases with differing risk will have differing predictive values.

The predictive value positive for all stages of disease is greatest, and essentially equivalent, for 2-EIA and STTT as compared with other testing approaches. In view of the technical and temporal (duration of illness) constraints of Western immunoblot in STTT, 2-EIA seems to offer equivalent and simplified performance.

The predictive negative value is high in cases of low pretest probability for all stages of disease. Thus, a negative result in these situations essentially rules out disease. By contrast, the negative predictive value is poor for early disease cases with high pretest probability. Under these circumstances, a convalescent serology is warranted. However, in latter stage illness suspicion the predictive value negative increases sharply for all tests and in all but the highest pretest probability (>80%) indicates an alternate diagnosis. The predictive value negative for the 2-EIA approach is equivalent or better than the STTT in all stages of illness.

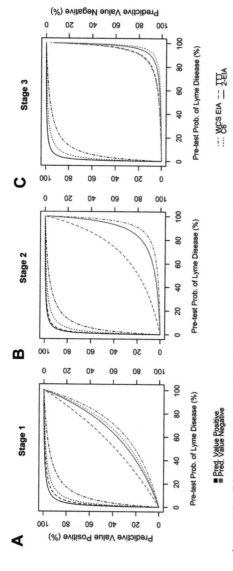

Fig. 1. Predictive value positive (*blue*) and negative (*red*) for the 4 diagnostic assays as a function of pretest probability (Prob.). (*A*) Stage 1. (*B*) Stage 2. (*C*) Stage 3. Lefthand axes mark the scale for predictive (Pred.) value positive, and righthand axes mark the scale for predictive value negative. Line types indicated in the legend identify the assays. WCS EIA, whole-cell-sonicate enzyme immunoassay.

TESTING FOR INFECTIONS ACQUIRED OUTSIDE NORTH AMERICA

Lyme disease infections acquired in the United States have been limited to *B burgdorferi* ss, whereas those in Europe include *B garinii*, *B afzelii*, and *B burgdorferi* ss. In general, antibody responses to infection with European genospecies causing Lyme borreliosis are of lower titer and to fewer antigens than those in the United States. A 2-tier serology algorithm similar to that in the United States is also recommended in Europe.[53] However, the number of bands required for positive IgM and IgG Western immunoblots by the European criteria are less than those required by US criteria. Several studies have assessed the sensitivity and specificity of US and European 2-tier testing criteria among patients with disease acquired in both regions.[38,54] As might be expected, sensitivity of the US STTT for patients with disease acquired Europe is less (52%) than that of European tests (81%).[38] Use of the C6 assay (licensed in both the United States and Europe) or a WCS-EIA followed by a C6 assay for European acquired disease demonstrated sensitivities of 88% and 84%, respectively.[38] Both of these approaches display very high specificity.

SUMMARY

Serology has been the mainstay of laboratory confirmation of Lyme borreliosis since direct detection of *B burgdorferi* has limited application. Since STTT for serology was put into common use in the mid 1990s, standardization and performance have improved. Although STTT detection of early, localized infection is poor, that of late disease is very good. Fortunately, the best indicator of stage 1 early infection, EM, is presented in the majority of US cases and when recognized in a relevant epidemiologic setting should prompt treatment without testing. Clinical and epidemiologic correlates of infection should be assessed carefully before ordering STTT and for evaluation of its results. Under these conditions, STTT has great value in the confirmation of extracutaneous stages of infection in the context of significant epidemiologic risk. Recent efforts to simplify serologic testing include use of recombinant antigens and alternatives to STTT. Further, these developments promise to improve performance, particularly in early disease detection.

SELF-ASSESSMENT

1. Skipping first-tier testing does not compromise test specificity because second-tier Western immunoblots are more specific than first tier EIAs.
   A. True
   B. False
2. IgG Western immunoblot reactivity is expected in cases with 4 or more weeks of duration.
   A. True
   B. False
3. Reactivity to any band in IgG or IgM Western immunoblots is indicative of exposure to *B burgdorferi*.
   A. True
   B. False
4. Positive 2-tier serology is considered confirmatory of active infection.
   A. True
   B. False
5. Western immunoblot enables distinction of reactivity to specific antigens that is not possible in whole cell lysate EIAs.

A. True
B. False

6. Assessing the pretest likelihood infection will help the physician to determine the value of testing and the probability that test results are true.
A. True
B. False

7. Clinical and epidemiologic correlates of infection are both important in the decision to order serologic testing.
A. True
B. False

8. Patients with several days of EM duration should have a positive 2-tier result.
A. True
B. False

9. Patients with 1 to 2 weeks of localized cutaneous infection or multiple EMs are equally likely to be seropositive by 2-tier testing.
A. True
B. False

10. Testing of persons with European exposure risk of Lyme disease by US 2-tier testing is acceptable because the species causing disease are closely related.
A. True
B. False

Answers

Answer 1: (B) False.
Requiring an equivocal or positive first tier test improves the overall specificity of serologic testing.

Answer 2: (A) True.
Immunoglobulin class switching from IgM to IgG is expected in less than 4 weeks.

Answer 3: (B) False.
Many *B burgdorferi* antigens contain epitopes that are conserved or crossreactive with those of other organismal antigens.

Answer 4: (B) False.
Positive serology indicates exposure but not necessarily active infection; positive antibody profiles may persist for months after curative treatment.

Answer 5: (A) True.
Many antigens are resolved in Western immunoblot and distinct antibody reactivity is assessed. In whole cell sonicate EIA the sum reactivity to all antigens is measured.

Answer 6: (A) True.
The pretest likelihood ranges over logs of order and the probability of true test results is correlated with this metric.

Answer 7: (A) True.
Clinical and epidemiologic correlates are equally important and may not support each other.

Answer 8: (B) False.
The mounting antibody response to infection typically takes more than 1 week before it is detectable by current serologic assays.

Answer 9: (B) False.
Patients with multiple EMs have a more robust antibody profile than those with a single EM.

Answer 10: (B) False.

Individuals with exposure to European genospecies causing Lyme borreliosis typically have a reduced antibody response as compared with persons exposed to *B burgdorferi* in the United States. The use of US 2-tier testing for European exposure is insensitive.

ACKNOWLEDGMENTS

The author thanks Brad Biggerstaff (Centers for Disease Control and Prevention [CDC], Fort Collins, CO) for kindly plotting **Fig. 1** and its critical review.

REFERENCES

1. Burgdorfer W, Barbour AG, Hayes SF, et al. Lyme disease-a tick-borne spirochetosis? Science 1982;216(4552):1317–9.
2. Steere AC, Grodzicki RL, Kornblatt AN, et al. The spirochetal etiology of Lyme disease. N Engl J Med 1983;308(13):733–40.
3. Preac-Mursic V, Wilske B, Schierz G. European *Borrelia burgdorferi* isolated from humans and ticks culture conditions and antibiotic susceptibility. Zentralbl Bakteriol Mikrobiol Hyg A 1986;263(1–2):112–8.
4. Kelly R. Cultivation of *Borrelia hermsi*. Science 1971;173(3995):443–4.
5. Wormser GP, Nowakowski J, Nadelman RB, et al. Improving the yield of blood cultures for patients with early Lyme disease. J Clin Microbiol 1998;36(1):296–8.
6. Wormser GP, Bittker S, Cooper D, et al. Yield of large-volume blood cultures in patients with early Lyme disease. J Infect Dis 2001;184(8):1070–2.
7. Aguero-Rosenfeld ME, Wang G, Schwartz I, et al. Diagnosis of Lyme borreliosis. Clin Microbiol Rev 2005;18(3):484–509.
8. Samuels DS. Gene regulation in *Borrelia burgdorferi*. Annu Rev Microbiol 2011; 65:479–99.
9. Radolf JD, Caimano MJ, Stevenson B, et al. Of ticks, mice and men: understanding the dual-host lifestyle of Lyme disease spirochaetes. Nat Rev Microbiol 2012; 10(2):87–99.
10. des Vignes F, Piesman J, Heffernan R, et al. Effect of tick removal on transmission of *Borrelia burgdorferi* and *Ehrlichia phagocytophila* by *Ixodes scapularis* nymphs. J Infect Dis 2001;183(5):773–8.
11. Oosting M, Buffen K, van der Meer JW, et al. Innate immunity networks during infection with *Borrelia burgdorferi*. Crit Rev Microbiol 2014. [Epub ahead of print].
12. Wormser GP, McKenna D, Carlin J, et al. Brief communication: hematogenous dissemination in early Lyme disease. Ann Intern Med 2005;142(9):751–5.
13. Smith RP, Schoen RT, Rahn DW, et al. Clinical characteristics and treatment outcome of early Lyme disease in patients with microbiologically confirmed erythema migrans. Ann Intern Med 2002;136(6):421–8.
14. Shapiro ED. Lyme disease. N Engl J Med 2014;371(7):684.
15. Edlow JA. Erythema migrans. Med Clin North Am 2002;86(2):239–60.
16. Aguero-Rosenfeld ME, Nowakowski J, Bittker S, et al. Evolution of the serologic response to *Borrelia burgdorferi* in treated patients with culture-confirmed erythema migrans. J Clin Microbiol 1996;34(1):1–9.
17. Coleman AS, Rossmann E, Yang X, et al. BBK07 immunodominant peptides as serodiagnostic markers of Lyme disease. Clin Vaccine Immunol 2011;18(3):406–13.
18. Signorino G, Arnaboldi PM, Petzke MM, et al. Identification of OppA2 linear epitopes as serodiagnostic markers for Lyme disease. Clin Vaccine Immunol 2014; 21(5):704–11.

19. Centers for Disease Control and Prevention. Proceedings of the First National Conference on Lyme Disease Testing, Dearborn, Michigan, 1990. Centers for Disease Control and Food and Drug Administration, Washington, DC, November 1–2, 1990.

20. Bakken LL, Case KL, Callister SM, et al. Performance of 45 laboratories participating in a proficiency testing program for Lyme disease serology. JAMA 1992; 268(7):891–5.

21. Craven RB, Quan TJ, Bailey RE, et al. Improved serodiagnostic testing for Lyme disease: results of a multicenter serologic evaluation. Emerg Infect Dis 1996;2(2): 136–40.

22. Coleman JL, Benach JL. Isolation of antigenic components from the Lyme disease spirochete: their role in early diagnosis. J Infect Dis 1987;155(4):756–65.

23. Karlsson M, Mollegard I, Stiernstedt G, et al. Comparison of Western blot and enzyme-linked immunosorbent assay for diagnosis of Lyme borreliosis. Eur J Clin Microbiol Infect Dis 1989;8(10):871–7.

24. Aguero-Rosenfeld ME, Nowakowski J, McKenna DF, et al. Serodiagnosis in early Lyme disease. J Clin Microbiol 1993;31(12):3090–5.

25. Dressler F, Whalen JA, Reinhardt BN, et al. Western blotting in the serodiagnosis of Lyme disease. J Infect Dis 1993;167(2):392–400.

26. Engstrom SM, Shoop E, Johnson RC. Immunoblot interpretation criteria for serodiagnosis of early Lyme disease. J Clin Microbiol 1995;33(2):419–27.

27. Johnson BJ, Robbins KE, Bailey RE, et al. Serodiagnosis of Lyme disease: accuracy of a two-step approach using a flagella-based ELISA and immunoblotting. J Infect Dis 1996;174(2):346–53.

28. Centers for Disease Control and Prevention. Proceedings of the Second National Conference on Serological Diagnosis of Lyme Disease, Dearborn, Michigan, 1995. Association of State and Territorial Public Health Laboratory Directors and the Centers for Disease Control and Prevention, Washington, October 27–29, 1994.

29. Centers for Disease Control and Prevention. Recommendations for test performance and interpretation from the second national conference on serologic diagnosis of Lyme disease. MMWR Morb Mortal Wkly Rep 1995;44:590–1.

30. College of American Pathologist. Tick-transmitted disease survey TTD-B. Northfield (IL): College of American Pathologist; 2009.

31. Steere AC, Coburn J, Glickstein L. The emergence of Lyme disease. J Clin Invest 2004;113(8):1093–101.

32. Shapiro ED. Clinical practice. Lyme disease. N Engl J Med 2014;370(18): 1724–31.

33. Steere AC, McHugh G, Damle N, et al. Prospective study of serologic tests for Lyme disease. Clin Infect Dis 2008;47(2):188–95.

34. Wormser GP, Liveris D, Hanincova K, et al. Effect of Borrelia burgdorferi genotype on the sensitivity of C6 and 2-tier testing in North American patients with culture-confirmed Lyme disease. Clin Infect Dis 2008;47(7):910–4.

35. Wormser GP, Nowakowski J, Nadelman RB, et al. Impact of clinical variables on Borrelia burgdorferi-specific antibody seropositivity in acute-phase sera from patients in North America with culture-confirmed early Lyme disease. Clin Vaccine Immunol 2008;15(10):1519–22.

36. Branda JA, Aguero-Rosenfeld ME, Ferraro MJ, et al. 2-tiered antibody testing for early and late Lyme disease using only an immunoglobulin G blot with the addition of a VlsE band as the second-tier test. Clin Infect Dis 2010;50(1):20–6.

37. Branda JA, Linskey K, Kim YA, et al. Two-tiered antibody testing for Lyme disease with use of 2 enzyme immunoassays, a whole-cell sonicate enzyme

immunoassay followed by a VlsE C6 peptide enzyme immunoassay. Clin Infect Dis 2011;53(6):541–7.

38. Branda JA, Strle F, Strle K, et al. Performance of United States serologic assays in the diagnosis of Lyme borreliosis acquired in Europe. Clin Infect Dis 2013;57(3): 333–40.

39. Wormser GP, Schriefer M, Aguero-Rosenfeld ME, et al. Single-tier testing with the C6 peptide ELISA kit compared with two-tier testing for Lyme disease. Diagn Microbiol Infect Dis 2013;75(1):9–15.

40. Nadelman RB, Wormser GP. Lyme borreliosis. Lancet 1998;352(9127):557–65.

41. Steere AC, Sikand VK, Meurice F, et al. Vaccination against Lyme disease with recombinant *Borrelia burgdorferi* outer-surface lipoprotein A with adjuvant. Lyme Disease Vaccine Study Group. N Engl J Med 1998;339(4):209–15.

42. Massarotti EM, Luger SW, Rahn DW, et al. Treatment of early Lyme disease. Am J Med 1992;92(4):396–403.

43. Bacon RM, Biggerstaff BJ, Schriefer ME, et al. Serodiagnosis of Lyme disease by kinetic enzyme-linked immunosorbent assay using recombinant VlsE1 or peptide antigens of *Borrelia burgdorferi* compared with 2-tiered testing using whole-cell lysates. J Infect Dis 2003;187(8):1187–99.

44. Greer DM, Schaefer PW, Plotkin SR, et al. Case records of the Massachusetts General Hospital. Case 11-2007. A 59-year-old man with neck pain, weakness in the arms, and cranial-nerve palsies. N Engl J Med 2007;356(15):1561–70.

45. Zhang JR, Hardham JM, Barbour AG, et al. Antigenic variation in Lyme disease borreliae by promiscuous recombination of VMP-like sequence cassettes. Cell 1997;89(2):275–85.

46. Liang FT, Steere AC, Marques AR, et al. Sensitive and specific serodiagnosis of Lyme disease by enzyme-linked immunosorbent assay with a peptide based on an immunodominant conserved region of *Borrelia burgdorferi* vlsE. J Clin Microbiol 1999;37(12):3990–6.

47. Wormser GP, Levin A, Soman S, et al. Comparative cost-effectiveness of two-tiered testing strategies for serodiagnosis of Lyme disease with noncutaneous manifestations. J Clin Microbiol 2013;51(12):4045–9.

48. Molins CR, Sexton C, Young JW, et al. Collection and characterization of samples for establishment of a serum repository for Lyme disease diagnostic test development and evaluation. J Clin Microbiol 2014;52(10):3755–62.

49. Tugwell P, Dennis DT, Weinstein A, et al. Laboratory evaluation in the diagnosis of Lyme disease. Ann Intern Med 1997;127(12):1109–23.

50. Lantos PM, Branda JA, Boggan JC, et al. Poor positive predictive value of Lyme disease serologic testing in an area of low disease incidence. Clin Infect Dis 2015. [Epub ahead of print].

51. Pepin KM, Eisen RJ, Mead PS, et al. Geographic variation in the relationship between human Lyme disease incidence and density of infected host-seeking *Ixodes scapularis* nymphs in the Eastern United States. Am J Trop Med Hyg 2012; 86(6):1062–71.

52. Halperin JJ, Golightly M. Lyme borreliosis in Bell's palsy. Long Island Neuroborreliosis Collaborative Study Group. Neurology 1992;42(7):1268–70.

53. Wilske B. Microbiological diagnosis in Lyme borreliosis. Int J Med Microbiol 2002; 291(Suppl 33):114–9.

54. Wormser GP, Tang AT, Schimmoeller NR, et al. Utility of serodiagnostics designed for use in the United States for detection of Lyme borreliosis acquired in Europe and vice versa. Med Microbiol Immunol 2014;203(1):65–71.

Alternatives to Serologic Testing for Diagnosis of Lyme Disease

Kevin Alby, PhD, D(ABMM)[a], Gerald A. Capraro, PhD, D(ABMM)[b],*

KEYWORDS

- Alternative diagnostics • PCR • Culture • *Borrelia* • Lyme disease
- Erythema migrans • Lyme arthritis • Neuroborreliosis

KEY POINTS

- The gold standard for laboratory diagnosis of Lyme disease remains serologic testing; however, culture and molecular testing may have a role to play in specific clinical scenarios.
- Studies comparing culture versus molecular testing continue to demonstrate the superior performance of molecular testing.
- Polymerase chain reaction detection of *Borrelia* DNA demonstrates exquisite specificity, but sensitivity of this method can vary depending on the specimen tested and the phase of disease.
- Alternative diagnostic modalities for Lyme disease should only be used on patients who have a high pretest probability for Lyme disease and should only be performed by laboratories with expertise in this area.

Lyme disease, caused by certain spirochetal members of the *Borrelia* genus, including *Borrelia burgdorferi*, *B garinii*, and *B afzelii*, is a chronic debilitating illness characterized by an inflammatory reaction to the organism in human tissue following exposure to the *Ixodes* tick vector. The disease manifests in multiple stages,[1] from early, localized skin infections (erythema migrans [EM]), to disseminated infection (eg, spirochetemia, meningitis), and then to persistent infection (eg, Lyme arthritis, neuroborreliosis). Some patients do not manifest all stages of disease, making timely diagnosis and treatment of the disease difficult. Although there are multiple species of *Borrelia* that are known or suspected to cause Lyme borreliosis in humans, *B burgdorferi* is the only causative agent of Lyme disease in the United States.

Disclosure statement: The authors have nothing to disclose.
a Clinical Microbiology, Department of Pathology and Laboratory Medicine, Perelman School of Medicine, University of Pennsylvania, 3400 Spruce Street, 4th Floor Gates Building, Philadelphia, PA 19104, USA; b Clinical Microbiology and Diagnostic Virology Laboratories, Department of Pathology and Translational Pathobiology, Louisiana State University Health Sciences Center – Shreveport, PO Box 33932, Shreveport, LA 71130, USA
* Corresponding author.
E-mail address: gcapra@lsuhsc.edu

The diagnosis of Lyme disease can be made clinically based on symptoms presented by patients and a history of recent tick exposure or travel to a geographic area where the *Ixodes* tick vector is endemic. The gold standard for laboratory diagnosis of Lyme disease has historically involved the detection of antibodies specifically directed against the spirochete. The Centers for Disease Control and Prevention (CDC) recommend a 2-tiered serologic algorithm that includes screening for antibodies using an enzyme immunoassay (EIA) or an immunofluorescence assay (IFA), followed by an isotype-specific Western blot for positive or equivocal EIA/IFA specimens. Available serologic methods for diagnosis of Lyme disease are covered in a separate article by Schriefer in this issue.[2] The antibody response to *B burgdorferi* infection begins to increase at 2 to 3 weeks after infection and peaks at 6 to 8 weeks for immunoglobulin M and 4 to 6 months for immunoglobulin G. Because of this extended time frame, it is, therefore, necessary to develop new diagnostic methods for earlier diagnosis and appropriate treatment of Lyme disease. This article reviews the alternative diagnostic approaches to serology, specifically *B burgdorferi* culture, nucleic acid amplification tests, and others. Many of these assays are in development and not in routine use for patient care; however, as research tools, they have provided a better understanding of the disease process and present new potential for laboratory diagnostic methods.

CULTURE

The gold standard for identification of many bacteria remains bacterial culture. As a diagnostic modality, culture suffers from diminished sensitivity and increased turn-around time compared with serologic methods of detection. One of the biggest benefits of culture for *Borrelia* species is its improved specificity over serologic methods for the identification of *B burgdorferi* in patients with a history of prior Lyme disease, who may have residual antibodies from the previous infection. *Borrelia* species present a problem in that they do not grow using standard culture conditions. Therefore, specialized culture conditions have been created to allow for culture of this organism from clinical samples. Indeed, it was the development of these culture conditions that allowed for the definitive linkage between the spirochete that became known as *B burgdorferi* and Lyme disease.[3] In these early studies, citrated blood was added to optimized Kelly medium. Kelly medium had been used previously to isolate other *Borrelia* spp from patients with relapsing fever.[4] This medium has subsequently become known as Barbour-Stoenner-Kelly (BSK). There have been several additional modifications to BSK medium to try and improve culture outcomes.[5,6] The BSK-H medium described by Pollack and colleagues[6] became the standard media for the isolation of Lyme *Borrelia*. Importantly, the BSK-H medium reduced the variability that had been seen in previous formulations of BSK. This interlot variability impacted several characteristics of Lyme *Borrelia*, including growth, morphology, and antigenicity.[7] Additionally, BSK-H medium could be created using materials from a single commercial source, the first media for Lyme *Borrelia* that had this advantage.[6] Although not the primary method for diagnosis of Lyme disease, the availability of a standardized culture medium allowed for improved research of what is still a controversial and poorly understood disease. Cultures for Lyme *Borrelia* are typically liquid based and incubated at 30°C to 35°C for as many as 12 weeks under microaerophilic conditions.[5]

The sensitivity of culture varies greatly because of the difficulty in determining a gold standard as well as variation in comparator methods. For example, when compared with polymerase chain reaction (PCR) of skin biopsies collected from patients with classic EM, culture was shown to be more sensitive than PCR for the detection of *Borrelia* from blood specimens.[8] However, other studies have looked at the comparison of culture with PCR of the tissue in patients with classic EM rashes and demonstrate superior performance of the molecular method.[9] Further information about the design and utility of PCR assays in the diagnosis of Lyme Borrelia infections are discussed elsewhere in this review. Modifications to BSK and BSK-H medium have continued to be made over the last 20 years with varying degrees of success. One of the more recent modifications changed the media composition as well as introduced a unique culturing strategy.[10] In this study by Sapi and colleagues,[10] serum was inoculated into starter cultures containing the modified BSK-H medium. These cultures were then combined into larger long-term cultures. The investigators reported an increase in sensitivity to 94% for the detection of CDC-defined Lyme disease at 16 weeks. This rate was an increase from a 47% rate of detection at 6 days and an 83% rate at 8 weeks. Part of the increase in yield was attributed to several modifications made to BSK-H medium. These modifications included changing the concentration of rabbit serum to 12%, dithiothreitol to 100 µg/mL, and rifampicin to 0.5 µg/mL. Importantly, these results have been unable to be validated in other laboratories; subsequent studies have questioned the results of these findings, suggesting the possibility of contamination.[11] This circumstance has led the CDC to maintain its recommendation to use only Food and Drug Administration–approved tests to aid in the routine diagnosis of Lyme disease.[12] Another earlier observation that has been recently revisited is the interaction of B burgdorferi with the extracellular matrix.[13] B burgdorferi is capable of binding collagen in vitro and actually forming microcolonies during prolonged growth.[10] These organisms are difficult to dissociate from the collagen matrix, making assaying growth difficult. One approach that has been successful to circumvent this has been to disrupt the matrix using proteases and then use PCR for the detection of Borrelia DNA.[14]

ANTIGEN DETECTION

Because of the difficulties in establishing a reliable culture method for Lyme Borrelia, a variety of non–culture-based methods have been explored. One alternative for a non–culture-based method of detection is identification of Borrelia-specific antigens in a patient's sample. The detection B burgdorferi antigens in urine, blood, and other infected tissues has been described by Dorward and colleagues.[15] The investigators developed antisera against an 83-kDa vesicle associated protein purified from B burgdorferi cultures, which was able to detect this antigen in a variety of sample types from infected animals and humans. In the case of urine samples, this method was able to detect antigen in 38 of 39 samples from infected patients. This method uses electron microscopy, however, to detect the antigen/antibody complexes, limiting the utility of this assay for routine clinical diagnostics. More recently, efforts have been made to develop ways to concentrate B burgdorferi antigens in the urine. Hydrogel microparticles consisting of N-isopropylacrylamide-acrylic acid were used to sequester and concentrate B burgdorferi antigens approximately 100-fold.[16] Further work in this area may lead to a clinically useful antigen detection assay for the diagnosis of Lyme disease. Currently available rapid diagnostic tests for B burgdorferi are designed to identify specific antibodies to the organism and do not perform as well as traditional laboratory-based algorithms.[17]

ASSAYS TO DETECT CELL-MEDIATED IMMUNITY

Although the detection of pathogen-specific antibodies remains the gold standard method for determining if there has been an immune response against a particular pathogen, other changes in immune cells can also be used. Lymphocyte transformation or lymphocyte activation tests are one such group of tests. These tests use the development of a CD4 memory T-cell response to antigenic challenge. These specific CD4 cells can be transformed or induced to proliferate on stimulation with an antigen ex vivo. Cells are harvested from peripheral blood, washed, resuspended in culture medium, and subsequently labeled with an active label, such as a heavy amino acid, followed by introduction of the antigen of interest. If specific CD4 cells are present, they will react to the antigen and begin to proliferate, generating new cells that are labeled with the heavy amino acid. Alternatively, the cell culture supernatant can be queried for the production of cytokines in response to antigen activation. This approach has been applied to the detection of Borrelia with mixed results. Several studies have demonstrated the presence of Borrelia-specific CD4 T cells and the ability to stimulate these cells ex vivo.[18–20] However, these assays have also been shown to suffer from a lack of specificity, demonstrating equal reactivity in unexposed populations, such as healthy blood donors or newborns to those exposed to B burgdorferi.[21,22] Other immunologic assays that have been postulated to serve as a method of detection of Lyme borreliosis include cell counts of natural killer cells using the CD57 cell marker,[23] which have also been found to be nonspecific.[24]

NUCLEIC ACID AMPLIFICATION TESTS

Molecular assays for the detection of Borrelia spp from clinical material have been in development for many years but have not become the gold standard diagnostic modality. Although these assays have demonstrated high specificity, sensitivity has been lacking. This lack in sensitivity is likely caused by the lack of a true gold standard assay or lack of a standardized approach for comparison of the various methods under development. Additionally, nucleic acid amplification tests (NAATs) have shown a range of sensitivities based on the clinical illness studied. The molecular approach to laboratory diagnosis of Lyme disease may also be complicated by the recognition of multiple distinct species of Borrelia that have been associated with Lyme borreliosis in humans.[25] With international travel becoming increasingly common, the possibility exists that clinical laboratories may be asked to identify Lyme disease from patients whose infections are caused by Borrelia species not endemic to the local area. NAATs can, however, serve as an adjunct diagnostic modality alongside clinical findings and serologic testing and, depending on the specimen source, perform well in cases of acute disease.[26–29] Early in the course of infection, NAATs may serve to confirm the diagnosis when the antibody response is undetectable by serologic methods. In later stages of disease and in cases of suspected reinfection, particularly when serologic methods may not establish the diagnosis, NAATs offer high specificity.

As a diagnostic modality, NAAT performance has been as variable as the assay designs themselves. Most NAATs investigated for the detection of B burgdorferi DNA have used a variety of PCR techniques, including end-point PCR, nested PCR, and real-time PCR.[30–32] Some studies have used DNA sequencing or pulsed-field gel electrophoresis to discriminate among target genes and to separate different species of Borrelia.[33–38] In addition to the technology selected for these assays, the DNA targets for amplification have also varied. Borrelia species contain both chromosomal and plasmid DNA, and molecular assays have been investigated using a variety of targets from both types of DNA.[39–41] Assays designed to target plasmid-borne genes, such as ospA, ospC, or vlsE, are more sensitive than those targeting chromosomal flagellin or 16s rRNA genes,[42,43] likely because of the finding that Borrelia often shed plasmid-containing blebs, which allows for higher concentrations of plasmid than chromosomal DNA. However, it is now well recognized that these blebs disassociate from the spirochete and may persist in tissues and body fluids[42,44]; therefore, detection of plasmid DNA from these nonviable blebs may elicit false-positive results that do not necessarily reflect ongoing Lyme disease. Chromosomal targets usually occur as single copies; although targeting these genes may result in lower analytical sensitivity, these genes may be a better predictor of organism viability.[33,38,42,45–50]

The application of NAATs to the diagnosis of Lyme disease has been investigated, and the data show that there is no one-size-fits-all approach. Studies looking at a variety of clinical material show that some matrices are better than others for the direct detection of *Borrelia* DNA from clinical specimens. The performance of these specimens in NAATs depends on the stage of infection at the time of patient presentation.

Erythema Migrans

Skin biopsies can be collected from EM lesions as early as 3 days after tick exposure.[39,51] One study showed that detection of *B burgdorferi* DNA was better from fresh or fresh-frozen lesions compared with paraffin-embedded or formalin-fixed tissue[39] (70% vs 44%). An earlier study from Schwartz and colleagues[45] reported the sensitivity of PCR in skin lesions as 59%, whereas Nowakowski and colleagues[9] compared the sensitivity of various diagnostic methods, including culture of skin biopsies and blood, PCR on skin biopsies, and serologic testing, in patients with EM and concluded that the most sensitive of these was amplification of DNA from skin lesions (80.2%). As a comparator method, this study cited the sensitivity of culture as 51% and 45% for skin lesions and blood, respectively. A more recent study compared the sensitivity of 5 diagnostic methods, including culture and a variety of PCR assays, and reported that one or more of these tests were positive in 94% of the patients enrolled,[8] demonstrating the potential for PCR to be highly sensitive in patients with untreated EM.

Disseminated Infection

Blood and urine have been investigated as potential specimen sources for molecular diagnosis of disseminated Lyme disease. Utilization of blood specimens for molecular diagnosis has been plagued by the low and transient spirochetemia encountered during infection, which is likely caused by the tropism of *Borrelia* for tissues, such as the heart, joints, and meninges,[27,39,41,52,53] and inhibition of amplification by heparin and hemoglobin.[53] However, Goodman and colleagues[54] showed that the sensitivity of PCR detection during spirochetemia was 18.4%; but if patients displayed clinical signs and symptoms consistent with Lyme disease, the detection rate increased to 30.3%; in the case of multiple skin lesions, it increased to 37.5%. Another study elucidated a temporal connection between DNA detection and spirochetemia. Maraspin and colleagues[27] showed that spirochete DNA was more commonly detectable soon after a tick bite rather than in later stages of the disease. Given this potential for false-negative results, detection of DNA in later stages of the disease should be interpreted with caution and should be correlated with serologic findings indicating a specific anti-*Borrelia* antibody response.[55,56]

Synovial fluid and CSF have been used as specimens for the molecular diagnosis of Lyme arthritis and neuroborreliosis. In cases of Lyme arthritis, a positive PCR result from synovial fluid is highly sensitive for the identification of *B burgdorferi* DNA and may confirm the diagnosis.[26,39,42,44,57–59] Sensitivity and specificity of synovial fluid for the diagnosis of Lyme arthritis has an average of 78% and greater than 99%, respectively.[39] Lumbar puncture and subsequent submission of cerebrospinal fluid (CSF) is necessary for cases of suspected neuroborreliosis; however, PCR as a testing modality is confounded by a low number of spirochetes in CSF[53] and spirochetal affinity to myelin.[60] Therefore, negative PCR results cannot rule out CSF infection. The performance of PCR assays to detect neuroborreliosis is highest early in the disease.[39,61] One small study reported detection of B burgdorferi DNA in 7 of 14 (50%) CSF specimens from patients with early neuroborreliosis but only 2 of 16 (13%) specimens from patients with the disease lasting longer than 2 weeks.[51] Centrifugation of CSF may improve the detection of Borrelia DNA.[27,61] Although the specificity of PCR for the diagnosis of neuroborreliosis is high (>99%), overall, there is a significant lack of sensitivity for PCR detection of B burgdorferi DNA in CSF from patients with Lyme disease, with an average of only 19%. Of the specimens investigated for molecular testing, urine has the advantage of being the least invasive specimen to collect from patients; however, several studies have documented its poor performance because of both false-negative (PCR inhibitors) and false-positive (nonspecific amplification) results.[29,39,51,57] Therefore, urine is not a recommended specimen type for the laboratory diagnosis of Lyme disease.

Acute Versus Chronic Infection

Specimens collected from patients with chronic Lyme borreliosis have shown a distinct drop in clinical performance compared with those with acute infection. In cases of acute neuroborreliosis, PCR on CSF is positive for B burgdorferi in 10% to 30% of cases; however, in chronic neuroborreliosis, B burgdorferi PCR results are rarely positive.[62] PCR on synovial fluid is positive in 50% to 70% of patients with Lyme arthritis, but the recovery rate from patients with chronic Lyme arthritis in unknown.[48,63] Notably, no such decline in sensitivity was observed for PCR testing on acute skin lesions of EM and chronic skin lesions of acrodermatitis chronica.[64]

PCR detection of B burgdorferi DNA has the advantage of decreasing the time to diagnosis of Lyme disease. After tick exposure, low concentrations of B burgdorferi DNA can be detected[28,61,65] from skin biopsies, but this is not sufficient to demonstrate active infection.[41] Additionally, negative PCR results do not definitively exclude infection. PCR may, however, be useful in patients who fail to mount a specific immune response. The variety of specimens tested using PCR has shown usefulness depending on the gene targeted by the assay and the stage of the disease. Biopsy of skin lesions during EM has the highest sensitivity; however, PCR in this scenario would be unnecessary because the presence of EM is pathognomonic for Lyme disease. Synovial fluid shows high sensitivity for Lyme arthritis, whereas CSF is an appropriate specimen for the diagnosis of neuroborreliosis. In an effort to maximize PCR sensitivity, performing at least 2 PCR approaches in tandem may be considered.[66] Alternatively, laboratories may consider offering PCR testing on a variety of clinical specimens, alongside the education of clinicians regarding proper specimen selection given the clinical presentation of patients. This approach would, however, necessitate validation, continued verification, and proficiency testing for all specimen types. Individual laboratories would have to assess their patient population to determine if this approach would be cost-effective or if the appropriate course of action would be to refer this testing to an experienced reference laboratory with expertise in Lyme disease PCR.

SUMMARY

Laboratory diagnosis of Lyme disease remains a significant challenge. Although nonserologic methods may play an adjunct role for the diagnosis of Lyme disease, they are not useful as a primary screening test. As with many laboratory tests, Borrelia culture and PCR should only be used in patients with a high probability of infection based on clinical manifestations and an appropriate exposure history. Although serologic testing remains the gold standard diagnostic modality, use of these other modalities may have important roles, especially during acute infection before the development of a serologic response. For most patients with classic EM or other classic manifestations of Lyme disease, use of these alternative assays may complicate the diagnostic picture and will certainly add significant health care costs with no proven benefit. These assays are critical, however, as research tools to aid in our understanding of *Borrelia* infection. It is hoped that their continued development will lead to improved diagnostic performance and possibly new diagnostic options for this difficult to manage disease.

SELF-ASSESSMENT

1. Your laboratory wants to establish PCR as the diagnostic modality for patients with Lyme arthritis. Which of the following specimens would provide the highest sensitivity for this assay?
   a. Skin biopsy of an erythema migrans lesion
   b. Serum
   c. Cerebrospinal fluid
   d. Synovial fluid
2. *Borrelia* culture for diagnosis of Lyme disease can be performed using which of the following media/incubation conditions?
   a. BSK-H medium incubated at 35°C for 12 weeks
   b. Chocolate agar incubated at 35°C for 7 days
   c. McCoy cells incubated at 35°C for 12 weeks
   d. *Borrelia* agar incubated at 35°C for 12 weeks
3. What biological phenomenon of the *B burgdorferi* life cycle has been associated with false-positive detection of *B burgdorferi* DNA by PCR assays?
   a. Free DNA following cell lysis
   b. Flagellin subunits that break off from infected host cells
   c. Plasmid-containing membrane blebs that dissociate from the *Borrelia* cell
   d. Plasmid DNA that diffuses through outer membrane pores
4. A positive PCR result does not necessarily guarantee the presence of living organisms. Which of the following PCR targets is considered to be a better predictor of organism viability?
   a. 16s rRNA
   b. vlsE
   c. ospC
   d. ospA
5. Which of the following specimens has the least sensitivity for PCR diagnosis of Lyme disease?
   a. Synovial fluid
   b. Urine
   c. Cerebrospinal fluid
   d. Skin biopsy of an erythema migrans lesion

Answers
   Answer 1: d
   Answer 2: a
   Answer 3: c
   Answer 4: a
   Answer 5: b

REFERENCES

1. Steere AC, Coburn J, Glickstein L. The emergence of Lyme disease. J Clin Invest 2004;113(8):1093–101.
2. Schriefer ME. Lyme disease diagnosis: serology. Clin Lab Med 2015, in press.
3. Benach JL, Bosler EM, Hanrahan JP, et al. Spirochetes isolated from the blood of two patients with Lyme disease. N Engl J Med 1983;308(13):740–2.
4. Kelly R. Cultivation of Borrelia hermsi. Science 1971;173(3995):443–4.
5. Barbour AG. Isolation and cultivation of Lyme disease spirochetes. Yale J Biol Med 1984;57(4):521–5.
6. Pollack RJ, Telford SR 3rd, Spielman A. Standardization of medium for culturing Lyme disease spirochetes. J Clin Microbiol 1993;31(5):1251–5.
7. Callister SM, Case KL, Agger WA, et al. Effects of bovine serum albumin on the ability of Barbour-Stoenner-Kelly medium to detect Borrelia burgdorferi. J Clin Microbiol 1990;28(2):363–5.
8. Liveris D, Schwartz I, McKenna D, et al. Comparison of five diagnostic modalities for direct detection of Borrelia burgdorferi in patients with early Lyme disease. Diagn Microbiol Infect Dis 2012;73(3):243–5.
9. Nowakowski J, Schwartz I, Liveris D, et al. Laboratory diagnostic techniques for patients with early Lyme disease associated with erythema migrans: a comparison of different techniques. Clin Infect Dis 2001;33(12):2023–7.
10. Sapi E, Pabbati N, Datar A, et al. Improved culture conditions for the growth and detection of Borrelia from human serum. Int J Med Sci 2013; 10(4):362–76.
11. Johnson BJ, Pilgard MA, Russell TM. Reply to "no evidence for contamination of Borrelia blood cultures: a review of facts". J Clin Microbiol 2014;52:1804.
12. Nelson C, Hojvat S, Johnson B, et al. Concerns regarding a new culture method for Borrelia burgdorferi not approved for the diagnosis of Lyme disease. MMWR Morb Mortal Wkly Rep 2014;63(15):333.
13. Zambrano MC, Beklemisheva AA, Bryksin AV, et al. Borrelia burgdorferi binds to, invades, and colonizes native type I collagen lattices. Infect Immun 2004;72(6): 3138–46.
14. Wood S, Rattelle A. Increased DNA yield following enzymatic release of *Borrelia* from a collagen matrix in culture. Journal of Microbiology and Experimentation 2015;2(1):00037.
15. Dorward DW, Schwan TG, Garon CF. Immune capture and detection of Borrelia burgdorferi antigens in urine, blood, or tissues from infected ticks, mice, dogs, and humans. J Clin Microbiol 1991;29:1162–70.
16. Douglas TA, Tamburro D, Fredolini C, et al. The use of hydrogel microparticles to sequester and concentrate bacterial antigens in a urine test for Lyme disease. Biomaterials 2011;32(4):1157–66.
17. Smit PW, Kurkela S, Kuusi M, et al. Evaluation of two commercially available rapid diagnostic tests for Lyme borreliosis. Eur J Clin Microbiol Infect Dis 2015;34(1): 109–13.
18. Dressler F, Yoshinari NH, Steere AC. The T-cell proliferative assay in the diagnosis of Lyme disease. Ann Intern Med 1991;115(7):533–9.
19. Buechner SA, Lautenschlager S, Itin P, et al. Lymphoproliferative responses to Borrelia burgdorferi in patients with erythema migrans, acrodermatitis chronica atrophicans, lymphadenosis benigna cutis, and morphea. Arch Dermatol 1995; 131(6):673–7.

20. von Baehr V, Doebis C, Volk HD, et al. The lymphocyte transformation test for Borrelia detects active Lyme borreliosis and verifies effective antibiotic treatment. Open Neurol J 2012;6:104–12.
21. Zoschke DC, Skemp AA, Defosse DL. Lymphoproliferative responses to Borrelia burgdorferi in Lyme disease. Ann Intern Med 1991;114(4):285–9.
22. Roessner K, Fikrig E, Russell JQ, et al. Prominent T lymphocyte response to Borrelia burgdorferi from peripheral blood of unexposed donors. Eur J Immunol 1994;24(2):320–4.
23. Stricker RB, Winger EE. Decreased CD57 lymphocyte subset in patients with chronic Lyme disease. Immunol Lett 2001;76(1):43–8.
24. Marques A, Brown MR, Fleisher TA. Natural killer cell counts are not different between patients with post-Lyme disease syndrome and controls. Clin Vaccine Immunol 2009;16(8):1249–50.
25. Schrieffer M. Borrelia. In: Jorgensen JH, Pfaller MA, Carroll KC, et al, editors. Manual of clinical microbiology. 11th edition. Washington, DC: ASM Press; 2015. p. 1037–54.
26. Swanson SJ, Neitzel D, Reed KD, et al. Coinfections acquired from ixodes ticks. Clin Microbiol Rev 2006;19(4):708–27.
27. Maraspin V, Ogrinc K, Ruzic-Sabljic E, et al. Isolation of Borrelia burgdorferi sensu lato from blood of adult patients with borrelial lymphocytoma, Lyme neuro-borreliosis, Lyme arthritis and acrodermatitis chronica atrophicans. Infection 2011;39(1):35–40.
28. Ivacic L, Reed KD, Mitchell PD, et al. A LightCycler TaqMan assay for detection of Borrelia burgdorferi sensu lato in clinical samples. Diagn Microbiol Infect Dis 2007;57(2):137–43.
29. Kondrusik M, Grygorczuk S, Skotarczak B, et al. Molecular and serological diagnosis of Borrelia burgdorferi infection among patients with diagnosed erythema migrans. Ann Agric Environ Med 2007;14(2):209–13.
30. Morrison TB, Ma Y, Weis JH, et al. Rapid and sensitive quantification of Borrelia burgdorferi-infected mouse tissues by continuous fluorescent monitoring of PCR. J Clin Microbiol 1999;37(4):987–92.
31. Pahl A, Kuhlbrandt U, Brune K, et al. Quantitative detection of Borrelia burgdorferi by real-time PCR. J Clin Microbiol 1999;37(6):1958–63.
32. Pietila J, He Q, Oksi J, et al. Rapid differentiation of Borrelia garinii from Borrelia afzelii and Borrelia burgdorferi sensu stricto by LightCycler fluorescence melting curve analysis of a PCR product of the recA gene. J Clin Microbiol 2000;38(7):2756–9.
33. Liveris D, Varde S, Iyer R, et al. Genetic diversity of Borrelia burgdorferi in Lyme disease patients as determined by culture versus direct PCR with clinical specimens. J Clin Microbiol 1999;37(3):565–9.
34. Wang G, van Dam AP, Schwartz I, et al. Molecular typing of Borrelia burgdorferi sensu lato: taxonomic, epidemiological, and clinical implications. Clin Microbiol Rev 1999;12(4):633–53.
35. Wormser GP, Liveris D, Nowakowski J, et al. Association of specific subtypes of Borrelia burgdorferi with hematogenous dissemination in early Lyme disease. J Infect Dis 1999;180(3):720–5.
36. Seinost G, Dykhuizen DE, Dattwyler RJ, et al. Four clones of Borrelia burgdorferi sensu stricto cause invasive infection in humans. Infect Immun 1999;67(7):3518–24.
37. Iyer R, Hardham JM, Wormser GP, et al. Conservation and heterogeneity of vlsE among human and tick isolates of Borrelia burgdorferi. Infect Immun 2000;68(3):1714–8.

38. Lee SH, Kim BJ, Kim JH, et al. Differentiation of Borrelia burgdorferi sensu lato on the basis of RNA polymerase gene (rpoB) sequences. J Clin Microbiol 2000; 38(7):2557–62.

39. Aguero-Rosenfeld ME, Wang G, Schwartz I, et al. Diagnosis of Lyme borreliosis. Clin Microbiol Rev 2005;18(3):484–509.

40. Dumler JS. Molecular diagnosis of Lyme disease: review and meta-analysis. Mol Diagn 2001;6(1):1–11.

41. Schmidt BL. PCR in laboratory diagnosis of human Borrelia burgdorferi infections. Clin Microbiol Rev 1997;10(1):185–201.

42. Persing DH, Rutledge BJ, Rys PN, et al. Target imbalance: disparity of Borrelia burgdorferi genetic material in synovial fluid from Lyme arthritis patients. J Infect Dis 1994;169(3):668–72.

43. Zore A, Ruzic-Sabljic E, Maraspin V, et al. Sensitivity of culture and polymerase chain reaction for the etiologic diagnosis of erythema migrans. Wien Klin Wochenschr 2002;114(13–14):606–9.

44. Carlson D, Hernandez J, Bloom BJ, et al. Lack of Borrelia burgdorferi DNA in synovial samples from patients with antibiotic treatment-resistant Lyme arthritis. Arthritis Rheum 1999;42(12):2705–9.

45. Schwartz I, Wormser GP, Schwartz JJ, et al. Diagnosis of early Lyme disease by polymerase chain reaction amplification and culture of skin biopsies from erythema migrans lesions. J Clin Microbiol 1992;30(12):3082–8.

46. Lebech AM, Hansen K, Brandrup F, et al. Diagnostic value of PCR for detection of Borrelia burgdorferi DNA in clinical specimens from patients with erythema migrans and Lyme neuroborreliosis. Mol Diagn 2000;5(2):139–50.

47. Oksi J, Marjamaki M, Nikoskelainen J, et al. Borrelia burgdorferi detected by culture and PCR in clinical relapse of disseminated Lyme borreliosis. Ann Med 1999; 31(3):225–32.

48. Jaulhac B, Heller R, Limbach FX, et al. Direct molecular typing of Borrelia burgdorferi sensu lato species in synovial samples from patients with Lyme arthritis. J Clin Microbiol 2000;38(5):1895–900.

49. Kruger WH, Pulz M. Detection of Borrelia burgdorferi in cerebrospinal fluid by the polymerase chain reaction. J Med Microbiol 1991;35(2):98–102.

50. Lebech AM, Hansen K. Detection of Borrelia burgdorferi DNA in urine samples and cerebrospinal fluid samples from patients with early and late Lyme neuroborreliosis by polymerase chain reaction. J Clin Microbiol 1992;30(7):1646–53.

51. Lebech AM. Polymerase chain reaction in diagnosis of Borrelia burgdorferi infections and studies on taxonomic classification. APMIS Suppl 2002;(105):1–40.

52. Stanek G, Fingerle V, Hunfeld KP, et al. Lyme borreliosis: clinical case definitions for diagnosis and management in Europe. Clin Microbiol Infect 2011;17(1):69–79.

53. Cerar T, Ogrinc K, Cimperman J, et al. Validation of cultivation and PCR methods for diagnosis of Lyme neuroborreliosis. J Clin Microbiol 2008;46(10):3375–9.

54. Goodman JL, Bradley JF, Ross AE, et al. Bloodstream invasion in early Lyme disease: results from a prospective, controlled, blinded study using the polymerase chain reaction. Am J Med 1995;99(1):6–12.

55. Chmielewska-Badora J, Cisak E, Wojcik-Fatla A, et al. Correlation of tests for detection of Borrelia burgdorferi sensu lato infection in patients with diagnosed borreliosis. Ann Agric Environ Med 2006;13(2):307–11.

56. Molloy PJ, Persing DH, Berardi VP. False-positive results of PCR testing for Lyme disease. Clin Infect Dis 2001;33:412–3.

57. Reed KD. Laboratory testing for Lyme disease: possibilities and practicalities. J Clin Microbiol 2002;40(2):319–24.

58. Nocton JJ, Dressler F, Rutledge BJ, et al. Detection of Borrelia burgdorferi DNA by polymerase chain reaction in synovial fluid from patients with Lyme arthritis. N Engl J Med 1994;330(4):229–34.

59. Bradley JF, Johnson RC, Goodman JL. The persistence of spirochetal nucleic acids in active Lyme arthritis. Ann Intern Med 1994;120(6):487–9.

60. Rupprecht TA, Koedel U, Fingerle V, et al. The pathogenesis of Lyme neuroborreliosis: from infection to inflammation. Mol Med 2008;14(3–4):205–12.

61. Gooskens J, Templeton KE, Claas EC, et al. Evaluation of an internally controlled real-time PCR targeting the ospA gene for detection of Borrelia burgdorferi sensu lato DNA in cerebrospinal fluid. Clin Microbiol Infect 2006;12(9):894–900.

62. Wilske B, Fingerle V, Schulte-Spechtel U. Microbiological and serological diagnosis of Lyme borreliosis. FEMS Immunol Med Microbiol 2007;49(1):13–21.

63. Eiffert H, Karsten A, Thomssen R, et al. Characterization of Borrelia burgdorferi strains in Lyme arthritis. Scand J Infect Dis 1998;30(3):265–8.

64. von Stedingk LV, Olsson I, Hanson HS, et al. Polymerase chain reaction for detection of Borrelia burgdorferi DNA in skin lesions of early and late Lyme borreliosis. Eur J Clin Microbiol Infect Dis 1995;14(1):1–5.

65. Honegr K, Hulinska D, Beran J, et al. Long term and repeated electron microscopy and PCR detection of Borrelia burgdorferi sensu lato after an antibiotic treatment. Cent Eur J Public Health 2004;12(1):6–11.

66. Picha D, Moravcova L, Holeckova D, et al. Examination of specific DNA by PCR in patients with different forms of Lyme borreliosis. Int J Dermatol 2008;47(10):1004–10.

Lyme Disease Coinfections in the United States

Adam J. Caulfield, PhD, Bobbi S. Pritt, MD, MSc*

KEYWORDS

- Tick-transmitted infections • *Ixodes* • *Anaplasma* • *Babesia* • Deer tick virus
- *Borrelia miyamotoi* • *Ehrlichia muris*–like agent

KEY POINTS

- Emerging tick-borne pathogens transmitted by *Ixodes scapularis* ticks include *Anaplasma phagocytophilum*, *Babesia* species, deer tick (Powassan) virus, *Borrelia miyamotoi*, and the *Ehrlichia muris*–like organism.
- Improved surveillance measures are necessary to more precisely determine the burden and geographic distribution of *I scapularis* ticks infected with these human pathogens.
- Better availability of diagnostic assays is necessary to more fully understand the prevalence and clinical manifestations of these emerging infections.

INTRODUCTION

Lyme disease is the most commonly reported vector-borne illness in North America, with more than 30,000 confirmed and probable cases annually.[1] Based on recent estimates, it is likely that the actual number of infections is closer to 300,000 cases per year.[2] It is caused by infection with the spirochetal bacterium *Borrelia burgdorferi*, and classically presents with fever, headache, myalgias, arthralgias, and a targetoid rash at the site of the tick bite (erythema migrans).[3] Patients are typically responsive to antibiotic therapy, especially if administered during the early stages of disease; however, if localized Lyme disease is left untreated, symptoms may progress to more serious rheumatologic, cardiac, and neurologic manifestations.

In the United States, Lyme disease is most prevalent in the northeastern and upper midwestern states. *Ixodes scapularis* (the blacklegged or deer tick) is the principal vector of *B burgdorferi* transmission, with *Ixodes pacificus* (western blacklegged tick) contributing to cases along the Pacific coast (**Fig. 1**). During the past decades, the geographic range of these ticks has been expanding, placing larger areas of

Disclosures: None.
Division of Clinical Microbiology, Department of Laboratory Medicine and Pathology, Mayo Clinic, Rochester, MN, USA
* Corresponding author.
E-mail address: pritt.bobbi@mayo.edu

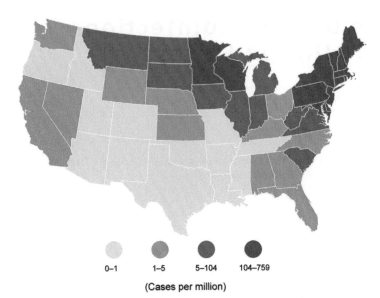

0–1   1–5   5–104   104–759

(Cases per million)

Fig. 1. Incidence and geographic distribution of Lyme disease in 2012. Data are not available for states in which anaplasmosis is not a notifiable disease. Based on statistics from the US Centers for Disease Control and Prevention (CDC). Available at: http://www.cdc.gov/lyme/stats/maps/interactiveMaps.html.

population at risk.[4] Although Lyme disease can be transmitted throughout the year, most reported cases occur during June and July because of the emergence of *Ixodes* nymphs in the spring and early summer. The nymphal stage ticks are small in size (2 mm), making them challenging to identify for removal.

As the incidence of Lyme disease increases, there are also greater possibilities for cotransmission of other pathogens carried by *I scapularis* and *I pacificus* ticks. These coinfections often present with nonspecific or overlapping symptoms and may thus complicate accurate diagnosis and treatment. Unless initially suspected by an experienced physician, patients with tick-borne coinfections may receive inadequate treatment and have a prolonged or complicated disease course. This article reviews the most common infectious agents transmitted by *Ixodes* species ticks in North America that have the potential for coinfection with *B burgdorferi* (**Table 1**), namely *Anaplasma phagocytophilum*, *Babesia* species, deer tick (Powassan) virus, *Borrelia miyamotoi*, and the *Ehrlichia muris*–like agent.

Anaplasma phagocytophilum (Anaplasmosis)

Introduction
The obligate intracellular rickettsial bacterium *A phagocytophilum* is the causative agent of human granulocytic anaplasmosis (HGA; previously known as human granulocytic ehrlichiosis).[5] It primarily infects granulocytes and multiplies within membrane-bound vacuoles to form microcolonies called morulae.[5]

Epidemiology
A phagocytophilum is transmitted by the same *Ixodes* ticks as *B burgdorferi* in the United States and is found in a similar distribution to Lyme disease (**Fig. 2**). Anaplasmosis was first recognized as a human disease in 1990 following the infection of a Wisconsin patient who died of a severe febrile illness after a tick bite; however, the

disease did not become reportable at the national level in the United States until 1999.[6] Since that time the annual rate of infections reported to the US Centers for Disease Control and Prevention (CDC) has steadily increased from 1.4 cases per million individuals in 2001 to 6.1 cases per million people in 2010, although current surveillance systems likely substantially underestimate the true incidence of A phagocytophilum infection in the United States.[7]

The highest incidence of anaplasmosis occurs among men greater than 60 years old within endemic areas.[8] A serologic survey of people with occupational risk for tick bites, such as forestry workers, determined that individuals with extensive outdoors exposures are at greatest risk for tick-transmitted Lyme disease and anaplasmosis coinfections.[9]

Clinical presentation

Typical clinical symptoms of HGA are nonspecific and include fever, chills, headache, myalgia, and fatigue arising 1 to 3 weeks following tick exposure. Unlike Lyme disease, rash is uncommon and is seen in less than 10% of patients. Most cases of HGA are mild and self-limited. However, severe manifestations may include respiratory failure, adult respiratory distress syndrome, peripheral neuropathy, rhabdomyolysis, acute renal failure, pancreatitis, and coagulopathies.[5] Risk factors for severe disease include comorbidities (eg, diabetes) and immune compromise.[10]

Laboratory diagnosis

Clinical laboratory findings commonly associated with HGA include thrombocytopenia, leukopenia, increased serum aminotransferase levels, and mild anemia.[5] A left shift with increased numbers of bands may also be seen. Morulae may be seen within neutrophils on peripheral blood films stained with Wright-Giemsa and other eosin-azure–type dyes (**Fig. 3**) and have been reported in up to 80% of cases during the first week of illness.[11,12] Finding morulae on peripheral blood smear is strongly supportive of anaplasmosis, but requires an experienced microscopist to differentiate true morulae from morula mimics such as overlying platelets, neutrophilic granules, and other inclusions.

Serologic assays are also commonly used for diagnosis. Indirect immunofluorescence antibody assays for detection of immunoglobulin (Ig) G class antibodies reacting with A phagocytophilum are considered the gold standard for serologic confirmation of anaplasmosis and are commercially available in the United States. However, antibodies are not usually detectable during acute disease because of delayed production by the adaptive immune response, necessitating testing of acute and convalescent sera, collected 2 to 4 weeks apart, for greatest sensitivity. A 4-fold or greater increase in titers between collections is considered diagnostic of anaplasmosis in the appropriate clinical setting. When paired sera are not available, a reciprocal titer of greater than or equal to 64 in a patient with a compatible illness is supportive (although not diagnostic) of anaplasmosis. Note that antibody response may be blunted if early therapy with doxycycline or other tetracycline-class antibiotics is administered. Furthermore, serologic tests may remain positive for months to years after acute infection and therefore cannot be used as evidence of cure.[13] IgM antibodies have lower specificities than IgG antibodies, and therefore positive IgM results should not be used as the sole method for diagnosis.[14] Note that there is significant cross-reactivity of antibodies to A phagocytophilum and Ehrlichia species.

DNA-based nucleic acid amplification tests, such as polymerase chain reaction (PCR), performed on whole-blood samples allow improved sensitivity and specificity compared with serologic assays during acute infection, with reported sensitivities of

Table 1
Prevalence of coinfecting pathogens carried by *I scapularis* ticks in the United States as determined by polymerase chain reaction

Location	Number of Ticks Sampled	Infection with:			Coinfection with:			Reference
		Bb (%)	Ap (%)	Bm (%)	Bb-Ap (%)	Bb-Bm (%)	Ap-Bm (%)	
Indiana	100 (a)	72	5	0	4	—	—	Steiner et al,[20] 2008
Maine	100 (a)	58	16	7	9	3	—	
Pennsylvania	94 (a)	52	1	0	1.1	—	—	
Wisconsin	100 (a)	35	14	0	8	—	—	
Maine	394 (a, n)	22.3	2.8	0.8	0.5	—	0.5	Holman et al,[76] 2004
Massachusetts	51 (a)	36	11	9	4	0	0	Telford et al,[77] 1996
Minnesota	419 (a)	37.5	11.7	2.5[A]	5	0.4[A]	0.4[A]	Stromdahl et al,[41] 2014
	348 (n)	25.9	7.5	3.3[B]	3.5	2[B]	0	
Wisconsin	201 (a)	25.9	3.5	0.6[C]	3	0	0	
	480 (n)	19.8	3.8	0.2[D]	1	0	0	
Pennsylvania	233 (a)	35.2	0.4	0[B]	0	0	0	
	300 (n)	19.7	1.7	0[E]	0	0	0	
New Jersey	100 (a)	43	17	5	6	2	2	Varde et al,[78] 1998
New Jersey	107	33.6	1.9	8.4	0.9	1.9	0.9	Adelson et al,[79] 2004
New Jersey	147 (a)	50.3	6.1	—	2.7	—	—	Schulze et al,[80] 2005

Location	Ticks							Reference
New Jersey	478 (n)	10.0	—	4.0	—	2.9	—	Schulze et al,[45] 2013
	610 (a)	45.2	—	8.2	—	6.2	—	
New York	100 (a)	52	53	26	—	—	—	Schwartz et al,[81] 1997
	73 (n)	26	21	5	—	—	—	
New York	3300 (n)	14.4	6.5	0.5	2.7	1.0	0.05	Prusinski et al,[19] 2014
	7904 (a)	45.7	12.3	6.3	2.5	1.5	0.6	
New York	4368 (n)	20.0	5.4	3.1	6.5	7.3	1.2	Hersh et al,[43] 2014
Pennsylvania	454 (a)	41.2	17.8	3.5	—	—	—	Courtney et al,[82] 2003
Pennsylvania	1363 (a)	47.4	3.3	2.0	3.5	1.5	<0.1	Hutchinson et al,[83] 2015
Wisconsin	89 (a)	11.2	7.9	2.2	—	—	—	Pancholi et al,[84] 1995
Wisconsin	636 (a, n)	—	3.8	—	—	—	—	Shukla et al,[85] 2003
Wisconsin: Kettle Moraine and Black River State Forests	383 (n)	34.2	7.8	3.4	—	—	—	Lee et al,[18] 2014
	365 (n)	22.7	3.0	2.5	—	—	—	
92 sites between Midwest and northeast states	5328 (n)	20.0	—	—	—	—	—	Diuk-Wasser et al,[86] 2012

Superscript letters indicate that the following numbers of ticks were tested: A, 242; B, 215; C, 175; D, 454; E, 271.
Abbreviations: (a), adult ticks; Ap, *Anaplasma phagocytophilum*; Bb, *Borrelia burgdorferi*; Bm, *Babesia microti*; (n), nymphal ticks.
Data from Refs.[18–20,41,43,45,76–86]

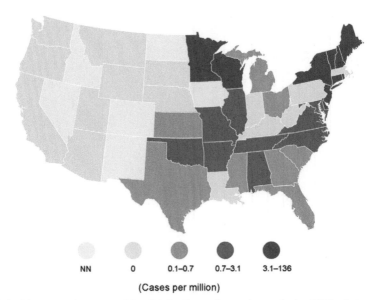

NN   0   0.1–0.7   0.7–3.1   3.1–136

(Cases per million)

Fig. 2. Incidence and geographic distribution of anaplasmosis in 2010. Data are not available for states in which anaplasmosis is not a notifiable disease (NN). More recently, cases of HGA have been reported from the Pacific Northwest (not included on the map). Based on statistics from the CDC. Available at: http://www.cdc.gov/anaplasmosis/stats/.

up to 95%.[15,16] There are currently no assays approved or cleared by the US Food and Drug Administration (FDA) and therefore existing laboratory-developed tests may vary in sensitivity and specificity. Testing is available through the CDC and select commercial reference laboratories and may be available as a component of multiplexed panels for other tick-borne pathogens.

Other methods for detection of *A phagocytophilum* include culture and tissue examination with use of organism-specific immunohistochemical stains. These techniques may be available at the CDC, but are not routinely used for clinical diagnosis.

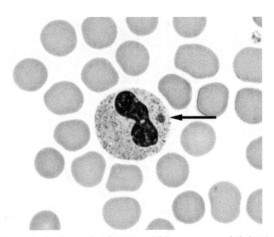

Fig. 3. Characteristic morula (*arrow*) of HGA within a neutrophil (Wright-Giemsa stain, original magnification ×1000).

Treatment and prognosis

Even though the mortality in humans is less than 1%, approximately 40% of patients diagnosed with HGA are hospitalized and at risk for secondary opportunistic infections.[7] Guidelines published by the Infectious Disease Society of America recommend empiric antibiotic treatment of all symptomatic patients suspected of HGA.[17] Doxycycline is the treatment of choice for patients with HGA or Lyme disease, alone or as a coinfection.[17] Given the potential for severe disease manifestations, doxycycline should be administered promptly in patients with suspected disease and not delayed pending laboratory testing, especially when serologic testing is used.[17] Prophylactic administration of doxycycline following tick bite and treatment of asymptomatic patients with positive *Anaplasma* serology are not recommended.[17]

Coinfection with Lyme disease

Vectors and reservoir hosts Several studies have examined the coinfection rates in ticks and small mammals in endemic regions. A recent study monitoring the infection status of ticks within 2 coniferous forests of Wisconsin determined that 26% to 35% of *I scapularis* nymphs were infected with *B burgdorferi*, whereas 3% to 9% were infected with *A phagocytophilum*.[18] Approximately 3% of *I scapularis* ticks examined were coinfected with both pathogens. A comparable study examined the infection rates of more than 11,000 ticks found in public parks of New York State's Hudson Valley Region.[19] Over a collection period of 4 years, the prevalences of *B burgdorferi* and *A phagocytophilum* were 14.4% and 6.5% among nymphs and 45.7% and 12.3% among adult ticks, respectively. The coinfection rates of nymphs and adults were 0.5% and 6.3%, respectively.[19] Similar studies have been conducted on questing tick populations from additional states, including Indiana, Pennsylvania, and Maine.[20–23] In a controlled laboratory environment, infection of *I scapularis* ticks with either *B burgdorferi* or *A phagocytophilum* had no impact on tick fitness or acquisition of the second agent from an infected host, and transmission of these agents to a new host occurred independently and with equal efficiency.[24] Rather than measuring the infection rates of tick vectors, a Minnesota study examined the disease burden of small mammal hosts that are heavily infested with *Ixodes* nymphs each spring. White-footed mice and eastern chipmunks were coinfected with *B burgdorferi* and *A phagocytophilum* at rates of 14% and 73% respectively.[25] These studies highlight geographic variation in infection rates among different tick populations and small mammals. The ongoing expansion of tick populations and their increasing rate of infection may lead to a greater incidence of human coinfections in the future.

Humans The frequency of humans with Lyme disease simultaneously coinfected with *A phagocytophilum* from various studies ranges from 2% to 10% based on the specific study methods and the case definitions used for HGA diagnosis. A study performed at New York Medical College specifically examined the impact of HGA case definition on coinfection rate. When a serologic definition (HGA IgG serologic titers >1:640) was used, the coinfection rate with *B burgdorferi* was 10%. However, when positive blood culture of *A phagocytophilum* was required for diagnosis of HGA, the coinfection rate was only 2%.[26] Similar coinfection rates have been reported from studies of Minnesota, Wisconsin, Rhode Island, and Connecticut residents.[23,27–29]

Babesia Species (Babesiosis)

Introduction

Babesiosis is an emergent hemolytic disease caused by protozoan parasites in the genus *Babesia*. The organisms are transmitted through the bite of infected *I scapularis* and *I pacificus* ticks and infect erythrocytes in a variety of hosts. Although more than 100 species of *Babesia* have been identified, only a few are thought to be pathogenic to humans. In the United States, *Babesia microti* is the predominant pathogen and is found in areas endemic for Lyme disease and HGA.[30] Less commonly, humans in the United States are infected with *Babesia duncani* or *Babesia divergens/B divergens–*like organisms (eg, MO-1 strain).[30]

Epidemiology

The first documented case of human babesiosis was reported in 1957 from a splenectomized Croatian herdsman,[31] whereas the first case from an immunocompetent individual occurred in 1969 in Massachusetts.[32] Over the past several decades, the geographic expansion of ixodid tick populations has led to an increased incidence of babesiosis (**Fig. 4**), with approximately 1000 to 2000 cases reported annually in the United States.[33,34] It remains largely unknown why infection of ticks and humans with *B burgdorferi* is more prevalent than infection with *A phagocytophilum* or *Babesia* species.

Most babesiosis infections are transmitted during the summer months, which correspond with the period of active feeding by *I scapularis* nymphs. The disease can be transmitted via blood transfusion, and is the most common transfusion-transmitted pathogen reported annually to the FDA. In rare cases, *Babesia* species can be transmitted across the placenta to the developing fetus.[30]

Clinical presentation

Following bloodstream inoculation with *Babesia*, sporozoites invade circulating erythrocytes and undergo asexual reproduction resulting in hemolysis, which releases heme and fever-inducing cytokines into the bloodstream. Most patients are asymptomatic or have mild, self-limited disease. When present, symptoms generally emerge following an incubation period of 1 to 4 weeks and consist most commonly of fatigue, headache, and myalgias. Complications include renal failure, acute respiratory distress, and

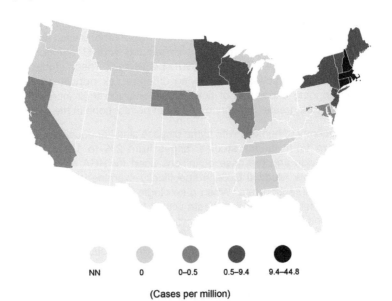

NN   0   0–0.5   0.5–9.4   9.4–44.8

(Cases per million)

Fig. 4. Incidence and geographic distribution of babesiosis in 2012. Data are not available for states in which babesiosis is NN. Based on statistics from the CDC. Available at: http://www.cdc.gov/parasites/babesiosis/data-statistics/index.html.

shock.[30] Risk factors for severe disease include asplenia, advanced age, and immune compromise.[35]

Laboratory diagnosis

Hemolytic anemia and thrombocytopenia are common laboratory findings. Babesiosis is principally diagnosed by microscopic identification of intraerythrocytic *Babesia* parasites using Giemsa-stained peripheral blood smears. Based on studies of malaria detection, this method is capable of detecting as few as 10 to 50 parasites per microliter of blood (approximately 0.0002%–0.001% parasitemia).[36] *Babesia* organisms appear as pleomorphic intraerythrocytic parasites that resemble the ring forms of *Plasmodium falciparum*, an important species that causes human malaria. *Babesia* can be distinguished from malaria parasites by their greater pleomorphism; lack of identifiable gametocytes; lack of brown-black hemozoin; and, when present, the tetrad arrangement of organisms (ie, Maltese cross)[30] (**Fig. 5**). The degree of parasitemia is commonly between 1% and 10%, but can reach high levels (ie, up to 80%) and cause life-threatening disease. Because the degree of parasitemia can be low during the early stage of babesiosis, at least 300 high-power microscopic fields should be examined. Note that the different human-infecting *Babesia* species cannot be reliably differentiated using solely morphologic criteria.

Molecular tests such as real-time PCR provide enhanced sensitivity compared with conventional blood smears and may allow determination of the infecting species.[37,38] The use of serologic assays for *Babesia* IgG antibodies may support the diagnosis of babesiosis, but these assays are primarily used for seroepidemiologic population surveys.[39] As with HGA, diagnostic antibody levels are not usually detectable during acute disease and therefore serologic testing is not reliable for detection of acute disease.

Treatment and prognosis

Most cases of babesiosis are mild and resolve on their own with treatment. Treatment is generally reserved for those with severe symptoms or that have risk factors for severe disease. Unlike Lyme and HGA, doxycycline is not an effective treatment of

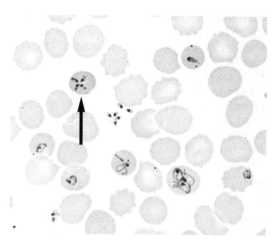

Fig. 5. Babesiosis caused by the *B divergens*–like parasite, MO-1. The intraerythrocytic parasites are round to elliptical and have bizarre ameboid forms, extracellular parasites, and frequent tetrads (*arrow*). The tetrads are not commonly seen in cases of babesiosis caused by *B microti*.

babesiosis. Instead, atovaquone and azithromycin are administered, with the alternative combination of clindamycin with quinine typically reserved for severely ill patients.[30] Critically ill patients and those with parasitemia loads of 10% or higher may also benefit from red blood cell exchange transfusion.

Coinfection with Lyme disease

Vectors and reservoir hosts There are several small studies examining the natural coinfection rate of B burgdorferi and B microti in I scapularis ticks. Because the methods of these studies are not standardized and represent different geographic regions, reported coinfection prevalence rates vary substantially, from 0% to 19%, for I scapularis ticks.[40–42] A large-scale survey of questing I scapularis ticks collected in Dutchess County, New York, determined that the prevalence of coinfection with B burgdorferi and B microti was significantly higher than predicted by chance based on the overall prevalence of each agent,[43] suggesting a possible synergy of infection.[44] This phenomenon has also been observed elsewhere.[45]

Humans In a study of patients with Lyme disease from southern New England, approximately 10% were coinfected with babesiosis.[46] Aside from individual case reports, there are few studies detailing the clinical outcomes of patients coinfected with Lyme disease and babesiosis. However, current evidence suggests that these patients have a greater number of individual symptoms with a prolonged duration compared with patients with Lyme disease alone. Coinfected patients were more likely to experience influenzalike symptoms, splenomegaly, anemia, and thrombocytopenia, which are not commonly seen with Lyme disease.[46,47] Because most babesia infections are subclinical, a delayed diagnosis may also contribute to the additional symptoms observed during a coinfection. There is no evidence that persistent long-term musculoskeletal or neurologic symptoms of Lyme disease are enhanced by coinfection with Babesia species.[48]

Deer Tick (Powassan) Virus

Introduction

Deer tick virus is a tick-transmitted RNA flavivirus that is classified as an evolutionary subtype (lineage II) of the encephalitis-associated Powassan virus. Lineage I (prototype Powassan virus) and lineage II (deer tick virus) share 94% amino acid identity and are antigenically indistinguishable in serologic assays.[49] However, they are transmitted by different species of Ixodes ticks and are maintained in discreet natural transmission cycles.[49,50] Lineage I is transmitted by Ixodes cookei and Ixodes marxi, which are found throughout the United States and rarely bite humans, preferring instead to feed on medium-sized mammals such as woodchucks and skunks.[51] In contrast, lineage II is transmitted by I scapularis ticks that are located in the upper Midwest and eastern United States and readily feed on human hosts. The association with I scapularis allows potential cotransmission of deer tick virus and B burgdorferi.

Epidemiology

Deer tick virus was first isolated from I scapularis ticks in 1997, the same year as the first reported case of fatal human deer tick virus encephalitis.[52,53] Since that time, only 4 cases of fatal tick-borne encephalitis have been linked to deer tick virus in the United States; cases have occurred in Canada, New York, and Minnesota.[53–56]

Clinical presentation

Neuroinvasive Powassan virus encephalitis cases are very rare, with only 36 cases reported from eastern Canada and the United States from 1958 to 2005, and approximately 70 total cases reported since 2012.[51,55] Most of these patients developed febrile encephalitis with acute onset of headache, confusion, and muscle weakness, with progressive neurologic symptoms. Following recovery from acute encephalitis, permanent neurologic sequelae generally persist. Cases of Powassan virus encephalitis caused by prototype Powassan virus (lineage I) and deer tick virus (lineage II) cannot be differentiated by clinical presentation.

Laboratory diagnosis

Diagnostic testing for deer tick virus is generally limited to state public health laboratories and the CDC, where serologic assays and reverse transcription PCR are performed for Powassan viruses. Molecular testing to differentiate prototypic Powassan virus from deer tick virus is typically not performed; instead, cases are classified base on the patient's exposure to *I scapularis* ticks and the local prevalence of deer tick virus. Most of the previously reported Powassan virus encephalitis cases attributed to prototype Powassan virus (lineage I) were diagnosed by serologic assays alone, so an unknown fraction may be attributable to deer tick virus (lineage II).[55]

Treatment and prognosis

As with other flavivirus infections such as dengue and West Nile virus, there is no specific treatment beyond supportive care for deer tick virus encephalitis. The case fatality rate following acute infection is approximately 10%, and permanent neurologic sequelae, including severe headaches and memory loss, persist in 50% of survivors.[57]

Coinfection with Lyme disease

Vectors and reservoir hosts At present, there are no studies that have specifically investigated the prevalence of ticks coinfected with *B burgdorferi* and deer tick virus. However, these agents share overlapping geographic distributions and both infect *I scapularis* ticks, making coinfection a plausible risk. In the laboratory setting, it was shown that *I scapularis* nymphs can efficiently transmit Powassan viruses to naive mice after only 15 minutes of attachment.[58] This enhanced transmission efficiency of deer tick virus compared with *B burgdorferi* may contribute to an increased prevalence of this emerging disease. Laboratory studies have established *I scapularis* as a competent vector of deer tick virus with transstadial and transovarial transmission rates of 22% and 17%, respectively.[58,59] Serologic studies suggest that, similar to *B burgdorferi*, white-footed mice may be the natural reservoir host of deer tick virus. Approximately 4% of mice collected from *I scapularis* endemic areas of Wisconsin and New England were seropositive for exposure to deer tick virus.[60]

Humans As a rare and recently described virus, diagnostic screening for deer tick virus infection among patients with Lyme remains limited, and therefore the incidence of coinfection with deer tick virus and *B burgdorferi* is unknown.

Borrelia miyamotoi (Relapsing Fever Borreliosis)

Introduction

B miyamotoi is a spirochetal bacterium in the genus *Borrelia*. Unlike *B burgdorferi*, it is classified in the closely related group of *Borrelia* that cause human relapsing fever.[61] The first case of human infection with *B miyamotoi* was described from Russia in 2011.[62] Infection has subsequently been identified in patients in the United States and Europe.[63–65]

Epidemiology

B miyamotoi seems to have a similar distribution to *B burgdorferi* in the United States, with a prevalence in *Ixodes* ticks of up to 10.5% in some regions.[66] Few well-documented human cases of *B miyamotoi* infection have been reported to date[63,64]; however, a recent large retrospective study of stored sera from blood donors in the northeast reported IgG antibodies to the GlpQ protein (found with infection caused by relapsing fever *Borrelia*) in 3.9% of 639 healthy individuals.[67]

Clinical presentation

As with other cases of tick-borne relapsing fever, the first human infections in Russia were associated with fever, chills, headache, myalgias, and (rarely) meningoencephalitis.[62] Limited data are available for cases of *B miyamotoi* infection in the United States, with only 3 confirmed cases with detailed clinical information. One case involved a highly immunocompromised 80-year-old woman from rural New Jersey who was evaluated following 4 months of progressive neurologic symptoms.[63] Spirochetes were observed in her Giemsa-stained cerebrospinal fluid, which also tested positive for *B miyamotoi* by PCR. Infection with *B burgdorferi* was specifically ruled out with negative serologic and PCR results from CSF. A 30-day regimen of intravenous penicillin G therapy correlated with a return in mental status to normal levels. The other 2 cases involved 61-year-old and 87-year-old men from Massachusetts and New Jersey, respectively.[64] These patients presented with acute-onset fever, thrombocytopenia, and leukopenia, and had increased liver enzyme levels. No rashes or attached ticks were discovered, but both patients reported regular recreational outdoors exposures. The diagnosis was achieved by testing whole blood using a PCR assay that can discriminate between *B burgdorferi* and *B miyamotoi*. Doxycycline was administered in both cases, and patients proceeded to full recovery.

Laboratory diagnosis

To date, agent-specific PCR assays have only been developed for research and epidemiologic purposes. Specific testing may be available through the CDC.

Treatment and prognosis

Reported cases of uncomplicated *B miyamotoi* experienced resolution of symptoms with doxycycline antibiotic therapy.[68] There are too few described cases to fully understand the outcomes of *B miyamotoi* infection in the United States.

Coinfection with Lyme disease

Vectors and reservoir hosts In a tick survey of 11 northern states, *B miyamotoi* was detected within questing North American *Ixodes* nymphs using PCR-based assays at a frequency of approximately 2%.[69] The same study found a 20% infection rate with *B burgdorferi*, with the coinfection rate of individual ticks with both *B burgdorferi* and *B miyamotoi* detected at the expected frequency caused by random chance.

Humans Given the recent discovery of *B miyamotoi* and limited surveillance, the prevalence and clinical significance of coinfections remain unknown. However, preliminary data suggest that Lyme coinfection is possible, with evidence of antibodies to *B miyamotoi* found in 9.8% of 194 patients with Lyme disease.[67]

Ehrlichia muris–like Agent (Ehrlichiosis)

Introduction

Ehrlichia is a genus of rickettsial Gram-negative bacteria that cause tick-borne illness in animals and humans. Following a tick bite, these obligate intracellular bacteria invade leukocytes or endothelial cells and lead to a febrile illness with headache, myalgias, and fatigue. Ehrlichiosis is the general term used to describe bacterial disease caused by at least 3 *Ehrlichia* species in the United States: *Ehrlichia chaffeensis*, *Ehrlichia ewingii*, and the more recently described *E muris*–like (EML) agent. *E chaffeensis*, and to a lesser degree *E ewingii*, are the main causes of ehrlichiosis in the United States. Both of these pathogens are transmitted by *Amblyomma americanum*, the lone star tick.[70] The EML agent was first identified in patients from Minnesota and Wisconsin in 2009 and was differentiated from other *Ehrlichia* species by molecular and genetic analyses.[71] The current cell types infected in humans is unknown. It has been detected only in *I scapularis* ticks and not in more than 6500 *A americanum* tested, suggesting that *I scapularis* is the vector of this emerging pathogen.[72]

Epidemiology

Unlike the other human pathogenic *Ehrlichia* species, the EML agent has only been detected in humans and *I scapularis* ticks from the upper midwestern United States. From 2004 to 2013, 69 human cases were detected by PCR out of 75,077 blood specimens tested.[73] The epidemiology features were similar to those of HGA and human ehrlichiosis: patients were predominantly male (64%) with a median age of 62 years (range, 15–94 years), and the peak onset of illness was in June and July. Most results (93%; 64 of 69) were detected among blood specimens from residents of Minnesota and Wisconsin, whereas the remaining 5 positive specimens were from patients living in North Dakota, Indiana, and Michigan. All patients reported likely tick exposure in Minnesota or Wisconsin, and the EML agent was not detected in 35,906 specimens submitted from patients in the 48 other states, suggesting that this new pathogen has a restricted geographic distribution.

Clinical presentation

With few documented cases and limited human testing, the prevalence of subclinical or asymptomatic infections is unclear. The most common symptoms among reported cases were fever, headache, and malaise, with laboratory findings significant for lymphopenia and thrombocytopenia. Of the 69 human cases detected, 13 patients were immunocompromised and 16 were hospitalized for 2 to 15 days (median, 4 days).[73]

Laboratory diagnosis

The most common laboratory findings among reported cases were increased liver function tests (78%), thrombocytopenia (67%), lymphopenia (53%), and anemia (36%).[73] Diagnosis has primarily been by real-time PCR analysis performed on blood samples from patients suspected of having a tick-borne illness. There are currently no commercially available PCR assays and testing is limited to reference and state public health laboratories in the upper Midwest. There are also no commercial serologic assays for the EML agent, but some cross-reactivity with *E chaffeensis* serologic tests has been observed. However, only 1 of 6 reported EML cases tested positive using *E chaffeensis* serology, suggesting that this is not a reliable method for diagnosis of acute disease.[73]

Treatment and prognosis

As with Lyme disease and anaplasmosis, the treatment of choice for ehrlichiosis is doxycycline.[71,74] Of the reported patients with EML infection, nearly all received doxycycline and all patients recovered.[73]

Coinfection with Lyme disease

Vectors and reservoir hosts The EML agent has also only been detected in *I scapularis* ticks sampled from Minnesota and Wisconsin (rate, 2.4%)[71] and not in *I scapularis* in northeastern, southeastern, or south central states.[72] It remains unclear whether this represents true geographic isolation of the EML agent to the upper Midwest or simply a lack of adequate diagnostic testing elsewhere. Further testing of tick and human specimens outside of Minnesota and Wisconsin would be useful for further defining the distribution of the EML agent in North America.

Humans In the largest study reported to date, 2 of 28 (7%) patients with PCR-confirmed EML infection tested positive for Lyme disease using either CDC-recommended 2-tiered serology algorithm or *B burgdorferi* PCR.[73,75]

SUMMARY

Several emerging agents, such as *A phagocytophilum*, *Babesia* species, deer tick virus, *B miyamotoi*, and the EML agent, can be transmitted by *Ixodes* species ticks and can cause coinfections with Lyme disease. The likelihood for human coinfection with multiple pathogens following a tick bite depends on the infectivity rate of both the *Ixodes* ticks as well as the mammalian reservoir hosts. Several studies have used PCR analysis to examine the prevalence of *B burgdorferi* and coinfecting pathogens. Although these studies establish an initial understanding, variability in tick collection methods, PCR assay parameters, and geographic sampling make the overall prevalence of coinfecting human pathogens among ticks difficult to establish. Therefore, there is a strong need for large-scale systematic studies to determine the distribution of pathogens within *Ixodes* ticks that continue to be an expanding burden on public health.

Clinically, possible coinfections should be considered in any patients who are diagnosed with Lyme disease, especially those who have unexplained leukopenia, thrombocytopenia, or anemia, or do not respond to antibiotic treatment of Lyme disease as expected. Continued and improved tick surveillance activities, diagnostic assay development, and clinician education will increase the understanding and awareness of Lyme disease coinfections.

SELF-ASSESSMENT

1. Which pathogen most commonly coinfects *I scapularis* ticks alongside *B burgdorferi*?
   A. *A phagocytophilum*
   B. *B microti*
   C. *B duncani*
   D. Deer tick virus
   E. *E chaffeensis*
2. Doxycycline is the recommended antibiotic for all of the following except infections with which agent?
   A. *A phagocytophilum*
   B. *B microti*
   C. *E muris*–like agent
   D. *B burgdorferi*
   E. *B miyamotoi*
3. Which pathogen has only been identified within *I scapularis* ticks in the upper Midwest region of the United States?
   A. *A phagocytophilum*
   B. *B microti*
   C. *E muris*–like agent

D. *B burgdorferi*
E. *B miyamotoi*
4. Asplenia is an important risk factor for severe disease with which of the following organisms?
  A. *B miyamotoi*
  B. *E muris*–like agent
  C. *A phagocytophilum*
  D. *B burgdorferi*
  E. *B microti*
5. Which of the following statements is true regarding deer tick virus?
  A. *I cookei* is the usual tick vector
  B. Infection is a form of tick-borne relapsing fever
  C. Human infection was first described in Russia
  D. It is a subtype of Powassan virus
  E. Doxycycline is the treatment of choice

Answers
  Answer 1: A
  Answer 2: B
  Answer 3: C
  Answer 4: E
  Answer 5: D

REFERENCES

1. Centers for Disease Control and Prevention. Notice to readers: final 2013 reports of nationally notifiable infectious diseases. MMWR Morb Mortal Wkly Rep 2014; 63(32):702.
2. Hinckley AF, Connally NP, Meek JI, et al. Lyme disease testing by large commercial laboratories in the United States. Clin Infect Dis 2014;59(5):676–81.
3. Borchers AT, Keen CL, Huntley AC, et al. Lyme disease: a rigorous review of diagnostic criteria and treatment. J Autoimmun 2015;57:82–115.
4. Kelly RR, Gaines D, Gilliam WF, et al. Population genetic structure of the Lyme disease vector *Ixodes scapularis* at an apparent spatial expansion front. Infect Genet Evol 2014;27:543–50.
5. Dumler JS, Choi KS, Garcia-Garcia JC, et al. Human granulocytic anaplasmosis and *Anaplasma phagocytophilum*. Emerg Infect Dis 2005;11(12):1828–34.
6. Chen SM, Dumler JS, Bakken JS, et al. Identification of a granulocytotropic *Ehrlichia* species as the etiologic agent of human disease. J Clin Microbiol 1994;32(3):589–95.
7. Dahlgren FS, Mandel EJ, Krebs JW, et al. Increasing incidence of *Ehrlichia chaffeensis* and *Anaplasma phagocytophilum* in the United States, 2000-2007. Am J Trop Med Hyg 2011;85(1):124–31.
8. Demma LJ, Holman RC, McQuiston JH, et al. Epidemiology of human ehrlichiosis and anaplasmosis in the United States, 2001-2002. Am J Trop Med Hyg 2005; 73(2):400–9.
9. Chmielewska-Badora J, Moniuszko A, Zukiewicz-Sobczak W, et al. Serological survey in persons occupationally exposed to tick-borne pathogens in cases of co-infections with *Borrelia burgdorferi*, *Anaplasma phagocytophilum*, *Bartonella* spp. and *Babesia microti*. Ann Agric Environ Med 2012;19(2):271–4.
10. Bakken JS, Dumler JS. Human granulocytic ehrlichiosis. Clin Infect Dis 2000; 31(2):554–60.

11. Bakken JS, Dumler S. Human granulocytic anaplasmosis. Infect Dis Clin North Am 2008;22(3):433–48, viii.
12. Schotthoefer AM, Meece JK, Ivacic LC, et al. Comparison of a real-time PCR method with serology and blood smear analysis for diagnosis of human anaplasmosis: importance of infection time course for optimal test utilization. J Clin Microbiol 2013;51(7):2147–53.
13. Bakken JS, Haller I, Riddell D, et al. The serological response of patients infected with the agent of human granulocytic ehrlichiosis. Clin Infect Dis 2002;34(1):22–7.
14. Brouqui P, Salvo E, Dumler JS, et al. Diagnosis of granulocytic ehrlichiosis in humans by immunofluorescence assay. Clin Diagn Lab Immunol 2001;8(1):199–202.
15. Chan K, Marras SA, Parveen N. Sensitive multiplex PCR assay to differentiate Lyme spirochetes and emerging pathogens *Anaplasma phagocytophilum* and *Babesia microti*. BMC Microbiol 2013;13:295.
16. Bakken JS, Aguero-Rosenfeld ME, Tilden RL, et al. Serial measurements of hematologic counts during the active phase of human granulocytic ehrlichiosis. Clin Infect Dis 2001;32(6):862–70.
17. Wormser GP, Dattwyler RJ, Shapiro ED, et al. The clinical assessment, treatment, and prevention of Lyme disease, human granulocytic anaplasmosis, and babesiosis: clinical practice guidelines by the Infectious Diseases Society of America. Clin Infect Dis 2006;43(9):1089–134.
18. Lee X, Coyle DR, Johnson DK, et al. Prevalence of *Borrelia burgdorferi* and *Anaplasma phagocytophilum* in *Ixodes scapularis* (Acari: Ixodidae) nymphs collected in managed red pine forests in Wisconsin. J Med Entomol 2014; 51(3):694–701.
19. Prusinski MA, Kokas JE, Hukey KT, et al. Prevalence of *Borrelia burgdorferi* (Spirochaetales: Spirochaetaceae), *Anaplasma phagocytophilum* (Rickettsiales: Anaplasmataceae), and *Babesia microti* (Piroplasmida: Babesiidae) in *Ixodes scapularis* (Acari: Ixodidae) collected from recreational lands in the Hudson Valley Region, New York State. J Med Entomol 2014;51(1):226–36.
20. Steiner FE, Pinger RR, Vann CN, et al. Infection and co-infection rates of *Anaplasma phagocytophilum* variants, *Babesia* spp., *Borrelia burgdorferi*, and the rickettsial endosymbiont in *Ixodes scapularis* (Acari: Ixodidae) from sites in Indiana, Maine, Pennsylvania, and Wisconsin. J Med Entomol 2008;45(2):289–97.
21. Steiner FE, Pinger RR, Vann CN, et al. Detection of *Anaplasma phagocytophilum* and *Babesia odocoilei* DNA in *Ixodes scapularis* (Acari: Ixodidae) collected in Indiana. J Med Entomol 2006;43(2):437–42.
22. Caporale DA, Johnson CM, Millard BJ. Presence of *Borrelia burgdorferi* (Spirochaetales: Spirochaetaceae) in southern Kettle Moraine State Forest, Wisconsin, and characterization of strain W97F51. J Med Entomol 2005;42(3):457–72.
23. Lovrich SD, Jobe DA, Kowalski TJ, et al. Expansion of the Midwestern focus for human granulocytic anaplasmosis into the region surrounding La Crosse, Wisconsin. J Clin Microbiol 2011;49(11):3855–9.
24. Levin ML, Fish D. Acquisition of coinfection and simultaneous transmission of *Borrelia burgdorferi* and *Ehrlichia phagocytophila* by *Ixodes scapularis* ticks. Infect Immun 2000;68(4):2183–6.
25. Johnson RC, Kodner C, Jarnefeld J, et al. Agents of human anaplasmosis and Lyme disease at Camp Ripley, Minnesota. Vector Borne Zoonotic Dis 2011; 11(12):1529–34.
26. Horowitz HW, Aguero-Rosenfeld ME, Holmgren D, et al. Lyme disease and human granulocytic anaplasmosis coinfection: impact of case definition on coinfection rates and illness severity. Clin Infect Dis 2013;56(1):93–9.

27. Mitchell PD, Reed KD, Hofkes JM. Immunoserologic evidence of coinfection with *Borrelia burgdorferi*, *Babesia microti*, and human granulocytic *Ehrlichia* species in residents of Wisconsin and Minnesota. J Clin Microbiol 1996;34(3):724–7.

28. Belongia EA, Reed KD, Mitchell PD, et al. Clinical and epidemiological features of early Lyme disease and human granulocytic ehrlichiosis in Wisconsin. Clin Infect Dis 1999;29(6):1472–7.

29. Steere AC, McHugh G, Suarez C, et al. Prospective study of coinfection in patients with erythema migrans. Clin Infect Dis 2003;36(8):1078–81.

30. Vannier E, Krause PJ. Human babesiosis. N Engl J Med 2012;366(25):2397–407.

31. Skrabalo Z, Deanovic Z. Piroplasmosis in man; report of a case. Doc Med Geogr Trop 1957;9(1):11–6.

32. Western KA, Benson GD, Gleason NN, et al. Babesiosis in a Massachusetts resident. N Engl J Med 1970;283(16):854–6.

33. Krause PJ, McKay K, Gadbaw J, et al. Increasing health burden of human babesiosis in endemic sites. Am J Trop Med Hyg 2003;68(4):431–6.

34. Centers for Disease Control and Prevention. Babesiosis surveillance - 18 states, 2011. MMWR Morb Mortal Wkly Rep 2012;61(27):505–9.

35. Homer MJ, Aguilar-Delfin I, Telford SR 3rd, et al. Babesiosis. Clin Microbiol Rev 2000;13(3):451–69.

36. Ochola LB, Vounatsou P, Smith T, et al. The reliability of diagnostic techniques in the diagnosis and management of malaria in the absence of a gold standard. Lancet Infect Dis 2006;6(9):582–8.

37. Teal AE, Habura A, Ennis J, et al. A new real-time PCR assay for improved detection of the parasite *Babesia microti*. J Clin Microbiol 2012;50(3):903–8.

38. Wang G, Wormser GP, Zhuge J, et al. Utilization of a real-time PCR assay for diagnosis of *Babesia microti* infection in clinical practice. Ticks Tick Borne Dis 2015; 6(3):376–82.

39. Krause PJ, Telford SR 3rd, Ryan R, et al. Diagnosis of babesiosis: evaluation of a serologic test for the detection of *Babesia microti* antibody. J Infect Dis 1994; 169(4):923–6.

40. Swanson SJ, Neitzel D, Reed KD, et al. Coinfections acquired from *Ixodes* ticks. Clin Microbiol Rev 2006;19(4):708–27.

41. Stromdahl E, Hamer S, Jenkins S, et al. Comparison of phenology and pathogen prevalence, including infection with the *Ehrlichia muris*-like (EML) agent, of *Ixodes scapularis* removed from soldiers in the midwestern and the northeastern United States over a 15 year period (1997-2012). Parasit Vectors 2014;7:553.

42. Piesman J, Mather TN, Telford SR 3rd, et al. Concurrent *Borrelia burgdorferi* and *Babesia microti* infection in nymphal *Ixodes dammini*. J Clin Microbiol 1986;24(3): 446–7.

43. Hersh MH, Ostfeld RS, McHenry DJ, et al. Co-infection of blacklegged ticks with *Babesia microti* and *Borrelia burgdorferi* is higher than expected and acquired from small mammal hosts. PLoS One 2014;9(6):e99348.

44. Dunn JM, Krause PJ, Davis S, et al. *Borrelia burgdorferi* promotes the establishment of *Babesia microti* in the northeastern United States. PLoS One 2014;9(12): e115494.

45. Schulze TL, Jordan RA, Healy SP, et al. Detection of *Babesia microti* and *Borrelia burgdorferi* in host-seeking *Ixodes scapularis* (Acari: Ixodidae) in Monmouth County, New Jersey. J Med Entomol 2013;50(2):379–83.

46. Krause PJ, Telford SR, Spielman A, et al. Concurrent Lyme disease and babesiosis - evidence for increased severity and duration of illness. JAMA 1996;275(21):1657–60.

47. Krause PJ, McKay K, Thompson CA, et al. Disease-specific diagnosis of coinfecting tickborne zoonoses: babesiosis, human granulocytic ehrlichiosis, and Lyme disease. Clin Infect Dis 2002;34(9):1184–91.

48. Wang TJ, Liang MH, Sangha O, et al. Coexposure to *Borrelia burgdorferi* and *Babesia microti* does not worsen the long-term outcome of Lyme disease. Clin Infect Dis 2000;31(5):1149–54.

49. Beasley DW, Suderman MT, Holbrook MR, et al. Nucleotide sequencing and serological evidence that the recently recognized deer tick virus is a genotype of Powassan virus. Virus Res 2001;79(1–2):81–9.

50. Kuno G, Artsob H, Karabatsos N, et al. Genomic sequencing of deer tick virus and phylogeny of Powassan-related viruses of North America. Am J Trop Med Hyg 2001;65(5):671–6.

51. Hinten SR, Beckett GA, Gensheimer KF, et al. Increased recognition of Powassan encephalitis in the United States, 1999-2005. Vector Borne Zoonotic Dis 2008; 8(6):733–40.

52. Telford SR 3rd, Armstrong PM, Katavolos P, et al. A new tick-borne encephalitis-like virus infecting New England deer ticks, *Ixodes dammini*. Emerg Infect Dis 1997;3(2):165–70.

53. Gholam BI, Puksa S, Provias JP. Powassan encephalitis: a case report with neuropathology and literature review. CMAJ 1999;161(11):1419–22.

54. Tavakoli NP, Wang H, Dupuis M, et al. Fatal case of deer tick virus encephalitis. N Engl J Med 2009;360(20):2099–107.

55. El Khoury MY, Hull RC, Bryant PW, et al. Diagnosis of acute deer tick virus encephalitis. Clin Infect Dis 2013;56(4):e40–7.

56. Birge J, Sonnesyn S. Powassan virus encephalitis, Minnesota, USA. Emerg Infect Dis 2012;18(10):1669–71.

57. Ebel GD. Update on Powassan virus: emergence of a North American tick-borne flavivirus. Annu Rev Entomol 2010;55:95–110.

58. Ebel GD, Kramer LD. Short report: duration of tick attachment required for transmission of Powassan virus by deer ticks. Am J Trop Med Hyg 2004;71(3):268–71.

59. Costero A, Grayson MA. Experimental transmission of Powassan virus (Flaviviridae) by *Ixodes scapularis* ticks (Acari: Ixodidae). Am J Trop Med Hyg 1996; 55(5):536–46.

60. Ebel GD, Campbell EN, Goethert HK, et al. Enzootic transmission of deer tick virus in New England and Wisconsin sites. Am J Trop Med Hyg 2000;63(1–2): 36–42.

61. Fukunaga M, Takahashi Y, Tsuruta Y, et al. Genetic and phenotypic analysis of *Borrelia miyamotoi* sp. nov., isolated from the ixodid tick *Ixodes persulcatus*, the vector for Lyme disease in Japan. Int J Syst Bacteriol 1995;45(4):804–10.

62. Platonov AE, Karan LS, Kolyasnikova NM, et al. Humans infected with relapsing fever spirochete *Borrelia miyamotoi*, Russia. Emerg Infect Dis 2011;17(10): 1816–23.

63. Gugliotta JL, Goethert HK, Berardi VP, et al. Meningoencephalitis from *Borrelia miyamotoi* in an immunocompromised patient. N Engl J Med 2013;368(3): 240–5.

64. Chowdri HR, Gugliotta JL, Berardi VP, et al. *Borrelia miyamotoi* infection presenting as human granulocytic anaplasmosis: a case report. Ann Intern Med 2013; 159(1):21–7.

65. Hovius JW, de Wever B, Sohne M, et al. A case of meningoencephalitis by the relapsing fever spirochaete *Borrelia miyamotoi* in Europe. Lancet 2013; 382(9892):658.

66. Wormser GP, Pritt B. Update and commentary on four emerging tick-borne infections: *Ehrlichia muris*-like agent, *Borrelia miyamotoi*, deer tick virus, heartland virus, and whether ticks play a role in transmission of *Bartonella henselae*. Infect Dis Clin North Am 2015;29(2):371–81.

67. Krause PJ, Narasimhan S, Wormser GP, et al. *Borrelia miyamotoi* sensu lato seroreactivity and seroprevalence in the northeastern United States. Emerg Infect Dis 2014;20(7):1183–90.

68. Krause PJ, Fish D, Narasimhan S, et al. *Borrelia miyamotoi* infection in nature and in humans. Clin Microbiol Infect 2015;21(7):631–9.

69. Barbour AG, Bunikis J, Travinsky B, et al. Niche partitioning of *Borrelia burgdorferi* and *Borrelia miyamotoi* in the same tick vector and mammalian reservoir species. Am J Trop Med Hyg 2009;81(6):1120–31.

70. Ganguly S, Mukhopadhayay SK. Tick-borne ehrlichiosis infection in human beings. J Vector Borne Dis 2008;45(4):273–80.

71. Pritt BS, Sloan LM, Johnson DK, et al. Emergence of a new pathogenic *Ehrlichia* species, Wisconsin and Minnesota, 2009. N Engl J Med 2011;365(5):422–9.

72. Pritt BS, McFadden JD, Stromdah E, et al. Emergence of a novel *Ehrlichia* sp. agent pathogenic for humans in the Midwestern United States. 6th International Meeting on Rickettsiae and Rickettsial Diseases. Heraklion (Greece), June 5–7, 2011.

73. Johnson DKH, Schiffman EK, Davis JP, et al. Human infection with the *Ehrlichia muris*-like agent in the United States, 2007-2013. Emerg Infect Dis, in press.

74. Dumler JS, Madigan JE, Pusterla N, et al. Ehrlichioses in humans: epidemiology, clinical presentation, diagnosis, and treatment. Clin Infect Dis 2007;45(Suppl 1): S45–51.

75. Centers for Disease Control and Prevention. Recommendations for test performance and interpretation from the Second National Conference on Serologic Diagnosis of Lyme Disease. MMWR Morb Mortal Wkly Rep 1995;44(31):590–1.

76. Holman MS, Caporale DA, Goldberg J, et al. *Anaplasma phagocytophilum*, *Babesia microti*, and *Borrelia burgdorferi* in *Ixodes scapularis*, southern coastal Maine. Emerg Infect Dis 2004;10(4):744–6.

77. Telford SR 3rd, Dawson JE, Katavolos P, et al. Perpetuation of the agent of human granulocytic ehrlichiosis in a deer tick-rodent cycle. Proc Natl Acad Sci U S A 1996;93(12):6209–14.

78. Varde S, Beckley J, Schwartz I. Prevalence of tick-borne pathogens in *Ixodes scapularis* in a rural New Jersey County. Emerg Infect Dis 1998;4(1):97–9.

79. Adelson ME, Rao RV, Tilton RC, et al. Prevalence of *Borrelia burgdorferi*, *Bartonella* spp., *Babesia microti*, and *Anaplasma phagocytophila* in *Ixodes scapularis* ticks collected in Northern New Jersey. J Clin Microbiol 2004;42(6):2799–801.

80. Schulze TL, Jordan RA, Schulze CJ, et al. Relative encounter frequencies and prevalence of selected *Borrelia*, *Ehrlichia*, and *Anaplasma* infections in *Amblyomma americanum* and *Ixodes scapularis* (Acari: Ixodidae) ticks from central New Jersey. J Med Entomol 2005;42(3):450–6.

81. Schwartz I, Fish D, Daniels TJ. Prevalence of the rickettsial agent of human granulocytic ehrlichiosis in ticks from a hyperendemic focus of Lyme disease. N Engl J Med 1997;337(1):49–50.

82. Courtney JW, Dryden RL, Montgomery J, et al. Molecular characterization of *Anaplasma phagocytophilum* and *Borrelia burgdorferi* in *Ixodes scapularis* ticks from Pennsylvania. J Clin Microbiol 2003;41(4):1569–73.

83. Hutchinson ML, Strohecker MD, Simmons TW, et al. Prevalence rates of *Borrelia burgdorferi* (Spirochaetales: Spirochaetaceae), *Anaplasma phagocytophilum* (Rickettsiales: Anaplasmataceae), and *Babesia microti* (Piroplasmida: Babesiidae) in

host-seeking *Ixodes scapularis* (Acari: Ixodidae) from Pennsylvania. J Med Entomol 2015. http://dx.doi.org/10.1093/jme/tjv037.

84. Pancholi P, Kolbert CP, Mitchell PD, et al. *Ixodes dammini* as a potential vector of human granulocytic ehrlichiosis. J Infect Dis 1995;172(4):1007–12.

85. Shukla SK, Vandermause MF, Belongia EA, et al. Importance of primer specificity for PCR detection of *Anaplasma phagocytophila* among *Ixodes scapularis* ticks from Wisconsin. J Clin Microbiol 2003;41(8):4006.

86. Diuk-Wasser MA, Hoen AG, Cislo P, et al. Human risk of infection with *Borrelia burgdorferi*, the Lyme disease agent, in eastern United States. Am J Trop Med Hyg 2012;86(2):320–7.

Relapsing Fever Borreliae
A Global Review

Sally J. Cutler, PhD

KEYWORDS

- *Borrelia* • Tick-borne relapsing fever • Louse-borne relapsing fever
- Argasid (soft) ticks • *Pediculus humanus* • Clothing lice • Epidemic relapsing fever
- Endemic relapsing fever

KEY POINTS

- Most relapsing fever borreliae are transmitted by soft ticks belonging to the *Argasidae* genera; these are rapid-feeding ticks, and their bites may go unnoticed.
- The epidemic member of this group, *Borrelia recurrentis*, is transmitted by the human clothing louse, *Pediculus humanus*.
- Most relapsing fever *Borrelia* are zoonotic, with the exception of *Borrelia duttonii* and *B recurrentis*.
- Relapsing fever borreliosis should be considered among individuals with a relapsing febrile illness and travel history to an endemic region, particularly when malaria is in the differential diagnosis.
- Most infections are successfully managed with penicillin, tetracycline, or doxycycline. The Jarisch-Herxheimer (JHR) reaction can complicate treatment.

HISTORICAL BACKGROUND

The term relapsing fever was first coined after an outbreak of relapsing febrile illness in Edinburgh, United Kingdom. Although Otto Obermeier revealed the infectious etiology of relapsing fever in 1868, fulfillment of Koch's postulates proved challenging because of the predilection of this spirochete for its human host.[1] This limitation prevented publication of his findings until 1873, when sufficient additional evidence was generated to substantiate a causative role for the spirochete. Mackie subsequently disclosed the role of the human clothing louse, *P humanus*, as the vector responsible for transmission of this infection in 1907.[2] During these times, epidemic louse-borne relapsing fever (LBRF) resulted in substantial mortality, particularly during situations of overcrowding and poverty that favored rapid spread of the organism, facilitated

Disclosures: The author has no disclosures to declare or conflicts of interest.
School of Health, Sport and Bioscience, University of East London, London E15 4LZ, UK
E-mail address: s.cutler@uel.ac.uk

Clin Lab Med 35 (2015) 847–865
http://dx.doi.org/10.1016/j.cll.2015.07.001   labmed.theclinics.com

primarily by the clothing louse vector. Massive outbreaks resulted in millions of cases throughout Africa and globally during World Wars I and II.[3]

Livingstone described another variant of relapsing fever in 1857, this time associated with soft tick vectors.[4] Both Ross and Milne and also Dutton and Todd independently established the role of ticks in transmitting this form of relapsing fever in 1904, with Dutton and Todd both becoming accidentally infected themselves while undertaking their research.[5,6] Dutton kept a temperature chart of his relapsing fever until he succumbed to the illness, with the infectious agent being named after him to reflect his contribution to the understanding of this infection. These researchers drew the parallel between this agent and its louse-borne variant, and their observations were recently substantiated by full genomic sequencing of both infectious organisms.

Subsequently, other *Ornithodoros* soft ticks have been identified as vectors for different species of relapsing fever borreliae. Most of these species seem to have adapted to a particular tick species, and consequently, many are named after their tick vectors (**Table 1**).

CLASSIFICATION

Classification of members within the borreliae was initially based on the type of tick species that serves as their vectors, with the *Borrelia burgdorferi* sensu lato complex transmitted by *Ixodes* species ticks (hard ticks) and the relapsing fever borreliae transmitted by ticks belonging to the *Argasidae* genera (soft ticks; **Fig. 1**). This rather simplistic division has been challenged with the finding that *Borrelia miyamotoi* and *Borrelia lonestari* cluster phylogenetically among the relapsing fever *Borrelia*, yet are transmitted by hard ticks. There are now 23 validated relapsing fever *Borrelia* species, although others are awaiting sufficient data to achieve such status, and many of these agents show a distinct preference for transmission by a specific tick vector species. *Borrelia recurrentis* is the notable exception being transmitted by clothing lice (*P humanus*). **Table 1** lists most of the currently accepted species, although several novel species have recently been described, including *Borrelia mvumii* in ticks from Tanzania,[7] *Borrelia microti* and other species from Iran,[8,9] *Borrelia turicatae*-like *Borrelia* in bat ticks from the United States,[10] and as of yet unnamed species from penguins in South Africa,[11] although the species status and potential virulence of this agent for humans remains to be established.

The taxonomic position of relapsing fever spirochetes is a matter of controversy. Application of discriminatory typing tools (see section on diagnosis and typing) has revealed clades within species such as *Borrelia hermsii*. Others have reported different subpopulations within *B duttonii*, with all of the cultivable isolates grouped into just 1 of 4 subtypes.[12] Conversely, 16S rRNA gene sequencing has underscored the similarity between some species.[13] These similarities have been corroborated by whole genomic sequencing, which suggests that the LBRF, *B recurrentis*, actually represents a degraded subset of *B duttonii*.[14] Sequencing of the closely related zoonotic *Borrelia crocidurae* that predominates in West Africa has further highlighted how conserved these 3 African species are, despite their profound differences in host preferences, severity, and arthropod vectors.[15] Based on their conserved genomic makeup, yet diverse ecology, the above-mentioned 3 relapsing fever *Borrelia* spp may best be considered as ecotypes of a single species.

MICROBIOLOGY

Members of this group have a characteristic Gram-negative helical structure with 3 to 10 coils and a length of 10 to 30 µm and a width of 0.2 to 0.5 µm.[16] Typical of this

Table 1
Relapsing fever group species, their vectors, and geographic location

Organism Name	Arthropod Vector/ Reservoir	Vertebrate Reservoirs	Clinical Infection	Geographic Region
B recurrentis	Pediculus humanus	Man	LBRF, human	Africa (formerly worldwide)
B baltazardii	Unknown	Unknown	TBRF, human	Iran
B crocidurae	Ornithodoros sonrai	Rodents	TBRF, human	West Africa
B duttonii	Ornithodoros moubata	Man	TBRF, human	Africa (Central, Eastern)
B hermsii	Ornithodoros hermsi	Rodents	TBRF, human, canine	Canada, Western USA
B hispanica	Ornithodoros marocanus; Ornithodoros occidentalis; Ornithodoros kairouanensis (formerly Ornithodoros erraticus[a])	Rodents	TBRF, human	Algeria, Morocco, Portugal, Spain, Tunisia
B latyschewii	Ornithodoros tartakowskyi	Rodents, reptiles	TBRF, human	Central Asia, Iran, Iraq
B mazzottii	Ornithodoros talaje	Armadillos, rodents	TBRF, human	Southern USA, Mexico, Guatemala
B merionesi	Ornithodoros costalis Ornithodoros merionesi	Rodents	Unknown	North Africa
B microti	Ornithodoros erraticus[b]			Africa, Iran
B parkeri	Ornithodoros parkeri	Rodents	TBRF, human	Western USA
B persica	Ornithodoros tholozani	Rodents, bats	TBRF, human, cat	Asia, Middle East
B turicatae	Ornithodoros turicata	Rodents	TBRF, human, canine, birds	USA, Mexico
B venezuelensis	Ornithodoros rudis	Rodents	TBRF, human	Central & South America
Nonhuman Relapsing Fever Group Species				
B anserina	Argas miniatus Argas persica Argas reflexus	Avian species	Avian borreliosis	Worldwide
B theileri	Rhipicephalus annulatus Rhipicephalus decoloratus Rhipicephalus geigyi Rhipicephalus micropus	Ruminants Horses	Bovine borreliosis	America, Africa Australia Europe

Abbreviation: TBRF, tick-borne relapsing fever.
[a] *Ornithodoros erraticus* represented a tick complex. Recent taxonomic molecular studies redressed the phylogeny suggesting that *O erraticus* sensu stricto is not an efficient vector for *Borrelia*.
[b] Molecular confirmation of *O erraticus* identity unavailable at time of writing.

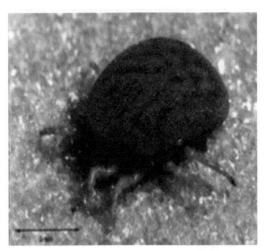

Fig. 1. *Ornithodoros moubata* tick.

genus, they have up to 30 flagellae residing within the periplasmic space between the outer membrane and protoplasmic cylinder. These endow a rapid gyrating motility to these spirochetes that can be seen using darkfield or phase microscopy of freshly collected specimens (see diagnostic methods section).

Porin proteins are found spanning the outer cell membrane and serve as a conduit for diffusion of low-molecular-weight compounds. The first of these described among relapsing fever spirochetes was p66.[17] Others have subsequently been described, such as Oms38, which appeared to be conserved between *B recurrentis*, *B duttonii*, *B hermsii*, and *B turicatae*[18] and shows homology with the DipA porin found among Lyme disease–associated borreliae.[19] Elucidation of such features will provide insights into the physiologic characteristics of these spirochetes and reveal potential targets for vaccine development.

The outer membrane lipid bilayer contains both lipidated and nonlipidated transmembrane proteins. Much attention has been focused on the abundant variable membrane proteins (Vmps) as these seem to be pivotal for rapidly switching between and surviving within the diverse environments of the arthropod vector and the mammalian host (see section on pathogenesis). Furthermore, these highly antigenic proteins are thought to contribute to binding of host factors, adhesion, and even tissue tropism.[20,21] Vmps have been extensively studied as they are subject to antigenic variation with an estimated recombination frequency of 10^{-4} to 10^{-3} per cell generation, providing a mechanism for evasion of the vertebrate host immune system. Such persistence mechanisms are likely to maximize the chances of transmission to uninfected arthropod vectors from infected vertebrates, thus providing a vital means of sustainability. They can generally be divided into 2 groups, small Vmps (also called vsp) with molecular weight ranging from 20 to 24 kDa or large Vmps (also called vlp) that typically range from 35 to 45 kDa.[16] The small Vmps have been likened to OspC of the Lyme disease spirochete, *B burgdorferi*; this has a key role in the transmission from arthropod to vertebrate host and establishment of early infection. Furthermore, expression of different small Vmps within *B turicatae* has been demonstrated to result in either central nervous infection (vspA) or blood-borne disease (vspB) with associated arthritis and myocarditis in a mouse infection model (see pathogenesis section). Expression of 1 small Vmp (vtp or vsp33) has been proposed as a tick-adapted variant. The large Vmps can be further subdivided into 4 groups (α, β, γ, δ) based on their sequence homologies. In the author's personal experience, human clinical isolates of B recurrentis and B duttonii expressed either small or large Vmps with no evidence of correlation.

The physiologic requirements of these microbes are poorly understood; however, their fastidious nature probably arises from their limited metabolic capabilities. This restricted biosynthetic repertoire necessitates the supply of amino acids, fatty acids, nucleotides, and enzyme cofactors from their surrounding environment, whether this is in their arthropod vector, the mammalian host, or complex growth medium (see section on diagnostic methods). Within the vertebrate host, the phenomenon of rosetting has been noted, and it is hypothesized that the borreliae are grazing to harvest essential nutrients such as purines from red blood cells.[22,23] Unlike B burgdorferi, the relapsing fever spirochetes contain a full set of purine salvage genes and demonstrate efficient acquisition and incorporation of hypoxanthine, the purine catabolic produce found within red blood cells, which might explain in part why these borreliae achieve higher blood densities than the Lyme disease spirochetes.

The genomic organization of these spirochetes differs from conventional bacterial dogma, as these microbes contain linear chromosomes with covalently closed telomeres and a combination of both circular and linear plasmids that comprise approximately 10% of the full genetic complement of these microorganisms.[24] Most essential house-keeping genes reside on the chromosome, whereas the lipoprotein genes tend to locate to the plasmids.[25]

Whole genome sequencing has been undertaken for 6 relapsing fever spirochetes, including B hermsii, Borrelia parkeri, B turicatae, B crocidurae, B duttonii, and B recurrentis (for further information see BorreliaBase[26]) and will provide a valuable resource to gain greater insight into the underpinning microbiological features of these organisms.[14,15] A striking observation arising from the project thus far has been the lack of any unique virulence features for B recurrentis when compared with the closely related B duttonii. As indicated earlier, this has led to the conclusion that rather than being a distinctive species, B recurrentis is instead a degraded subspecies of B duttonii that has become louse transmitted, although taxonomically it is still recognized as a separate species.

ECOLOGY AND TRANSMISSION

Most of the relapsing fever spirochetes are zoonoses with vertebrate reservoirs (see **Table 1**). In most cases, these reservoirs are rodents; however, bats, birds, and reptiles may also play a role in the environmental maintenance of these organisms.[27–30] Chipmunks have, for example, been noted as a significant reservoir species for B hermsii in the Sierra Nevada mountains of California. For B recurrentis and B duttonii, humans are the exclusive reservoir. Many consider the tick vector to also serve as a reservoir of infection for tick-borne relapsing fever (TBRF); this is facilitated by transstadial and, for some species, transovarial transmission of the spirochete between generations. In addition, these ticks have an impressive longevity during periods of starvation, allowing them to survive for many years while harboring the infectious spirochetes. The typical argasid tick life cycle is depicted in **Fig. 2**.

Some species that are grouped within the relapsing fever group have not been associated with human infection but instead cause febrile infection among food-producing livestock. These zoonotic agents include Borrelia anserina, the cause of avian

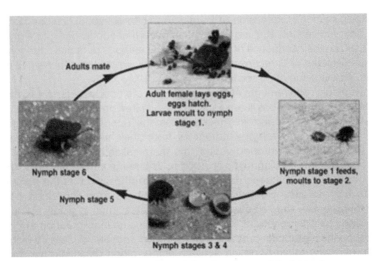

Fig. 2. Life cycle of *Ornithodoros moubata* ticks, the vector of *B duttonii*.

borreliosis transmitted by *Argas persicus* ticks; and *Borrelia theileri*, the agent of bovine borreliosis transmitted by *Rhipicephalus* tick species; *Borrelia coriaceae* transmitted to deer and cattle by *Ornithodoros hermsi* ticks among others.[31–34] It is highly probable that other livestock-related species exist[34,35] and that a plethora of other relapsing fever–related *Borrelia* persist among other as of yet undisclosed wildlife reservoirs.[11,36–38] Study of these borrelial species remains largely neglected.

Undoubtedly, poverty is a main contributory factor associated with increased risk for acquisition of a relapsing fever infection. **Figs. 3** and **4** portray some of these risk factors, including poor housing conditions and street beggars, which are at particular risk for relapsing fever. Both LBRF and TBRF have their greatest burden among those living in extreme poverty, who are often unaware of or unable to undertake the appropriate precautionary measures to reduce the risk of infection.[3] Those living in close proximity to ticks or vertebrate reservoirs are at additional risk for acquiring TBRF.[9,39] With increasing industrialization, urban homeless populations have seen an upsurge in clothing lice (**Figs. 5** and **6**), which could provide new clusters of disease if infected lice are introduced into permissive regions.[40] Another intriguing possibility for transmission and spread beyond the confines of clothing lice arises from the similarity between head and clothing lice exemplified by the overlapping phylogeny of clothing lice with cytochrome B clade A of head lice, formerly, "*P humanus* var *capitis*".[41,42] Specifically, this raises the question as to whether head lice could potentially serve as alternative vectors for *B recurrentis*. Individuals coinfested with both types of lice have revealed the presence of *B recurrentis* in head lice; however, the role of head lice in transmission requires further investigation.[43] This finding is further supported by the finding of other clothing louse-borne infections (*Bartonella quintana*) in head lice from individuals with no evidence of coinfestation with both ecotypes of *P humanus*.[44–46]

Occupational contact with tick-infested environments has resulted in clusters of TBRF infection. For example, among military personnel in Israel who used caves during training activities, approximately 6.4 cases of TBRF occurred per 100,000 individuals.[47] Similarly, environmental conservation workers in endemic areas are also at risk of infection. Imported cases have been encountered through migration and tourism

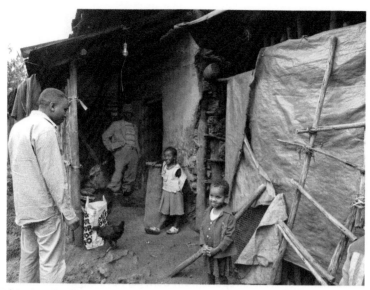

Fig. 3. Ethiopian dwelling.

where clinical suspicion in nonendemic regions may not be as heightened to exotic infections.[48–51] Several clusters and sporadic infections have also been traced back to vacation destinations in rural regions where intermittently used accommodations provide refuge for reservoir hosts and their associated tick vectors.[52]

EPIDEMIOLOGY

The relapsing fever spirochetes have historically been divided into Old and New World species; however, with improving phylogenetic tools, this division now seems rather artificial. The prevalence of tick-borne strains does show correlation with clearly demarked regions, as is particularly evident for African TBRF, and probably resulted from climatic conditions conducive for the specific tick vector[53]; this has not been

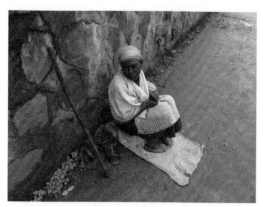

Fig. 4. Street beggar in Ethiopia.

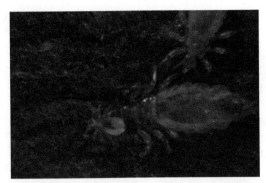

Fig. 5. *Pediculus humanus* clothing lice showing adult and subadult stages.

the case for the louse-borne *B recurrentis*, which was formerly worldwide but is now restricted to areas where clothing lice persist.[3,54]

What is becoming increasingly apparent, however, is the burden of relapsing fever infections occurring in endemic regions, many of which go undiagnosed or misdiagnosed as malaria.[4,55–57] Recent reports from Senegal have suggested that relapsing fever borreliae are the cause of approximately 13% of fevers presenting at local dispensaries, representing an alarming 11 to 25 cases per 100 person-years.[58] Studies of febrile patients in Morocco have suggested that 20.5% were due to TBRF.[59] Although not at such high levels, TBRF cases are more frequently being detected in the United States.[60,61] Given such data, despite consideration of relapsing fever as a neglected disease, it certainly should not be forgotten.

The epidemiology of LBRF has changed drastically over recent years, with the demise of this once worldwide infection correlated directly with the reduced level of infestation with clothing lice.[62] LBRF remains endemic in areas of extreme poverty such as in Ethiopia, at times spreading into adjacent regions, such as Sudan.

PATHOGENESIS

The pathogenesis of relapsing fever spirochetes is poorly understood, although the release of host cytokines is thought to play a major role. Production of interleukin (IL)-10 by the host can have a huge influence on clinical outcome demonstrating protection against microvascular injury and apoptosis of innate immune mediators but

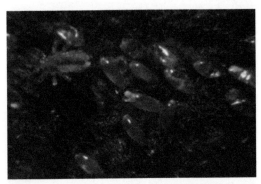

Fig. 6. *Pediculus humanus* clothing lice showing eggs cemented to clothing and recently hatched lice.

conversely can slow antibody-mediated clearance of spirochetes.[63] The borreliae, including those associated with relapsing fever, are neurotropic, and their sequestration within the central nervous system provides an ideal refuge from which new antigenic variants can reseed the circulatory system.[64] Animal experimental studies reported survival of borreliae months to years postinfection underscoring the ability of these spirochetes to reside within the brain.

Finally, the expressed surface Vmps play a pivotal role in pathogenesis. Some animal studies have shown correlation of particular clinical manifestations, for example, high blood counts versus neurologic infection, with the expression of different Vmps of the same B turicatae relapsing fever spirochete (see microbiology section).[65–68] Vmp proteins play a major role in the ability of these spirochetes to maintain high blood densities in their vertebrate host, sometimes reaching levels of 10^7 organisms per milliliter of blood; this is augmented through a gene conversion mechanism of antigenic variation that generates serotype switching and thus an intricate means of immunologic evasion.[69] This mechanism is further aided by the ability of borreliae to find serum factors such as factor H and factor H-like proteins.[70,71]

CLINICAL FEATURES

Transmission of TBRF follows the bite of an infected tick, whereas louse-borne infection follows inoculation of crushed lice or their feces into breaks in the skin such as through scratching. Unlike the transmission of Lyme disease borreliae that require attachment of their tick vector for an excess of 48 hours, transmission of TBRF borreliae is rapid and has been demonstrated in murine models to be possible in just 15 seconds using transmission of B turicatae by its Ornithodoros turicata tick vector. This transmission is largely a result of effective spirochetal colonization of the lumen of saliva-producing acini and possibly also the excretory ducts with spirochetes facilitating rapid and effective delivery of borreliae on initiation of tick feeding. Typically, argasid ticks feed nocturnally, with attachment times of 5 minutes to 2 hours being reported (average feeding time of approximately 20 minutes) and the tick taking up 2 to 6 times its original body weight in blood.

After an incubation period of 3 to 10 days, patients typically develop an abrupt onset of fever and chills. The duration of febrile episodes may vary, but the fever generally subsides in 3 to 5 days. This period is followed by an afebrile period that lengthens as the disease progresses interspersed by further febrile episodes. Individuals with LBRF may have 3 to 5 febrile episodes, whereas those with TBRF may have up to 13 recurrences of fever if left untreated. Each febrile episode correlates with a change in the surface Vmp antigens of the spirochete, and clearance is associated with development of a specific immunologic IgM response to the preceding borrelial serotype. The severity of these febrile periods generally reduces with time; however, organ involvement can complicate clinical recovery.

The most severe cases of disease are generally attributed to the human-adapted species, B recurrentis and B duttonii. Cases of LBRF typically present with fever, headache, hepatosplenomegaly, and joint and body pain and are often accompanied by abdominal tenderness, jaundice, and epistaxis.[72–74] Thrombocytopenia and renal impairment are common features following infection with B recurrentis. Major organ involvement of the brain, liver, lungs, and spleen result in a poor prognosis, with death associated with hepatic damage, cardiac failure, lobar pneumonia, subarachnoid hemorrhage, or splenic rupture. The factors that predispose to poor clinical outcomes are poorly resolved but are likely to involve the complex interplay between both host and microbial factors. The clinical manifestation of TBRF infections largely depends on the infecting *Borrelia* species and can range from a severe febrile disease similar to that described for LBRF as seen with *B duttonii* infection to a fairly mild febrile illness without associated mortality as seen for infection with *B crocidurae*. Some species are associated with particular clinical correlates, such as *B duttonii* and its adverse pregnancy outcomes, whereas epistaxis and jaundice are typical clinical features of *B recurrentis* infection. Historically, this clinical variability and differential severity has been used as a means of speciation through use of animal infection models (see diagnostic section), but the biological basis remains poorly resolved.

TREATMENT AND PROGNOSIS

Management of clinical cases is generally achieved with use of penicillin or doxycycline/tetracycline. Sometimes these are used in sequence, with penicillin being followed by doxycycline, as this might reduce the occurrence of potentially life-threatening Jarisch-Herxheimer reactions (JHR). This anecdotal observation has been substantiated not only by meta-analysis findings that showed more rapid clearance with tetracycline but also a higher risk of JHRs, whereas mortality rates were similar between the 2 treatment regimens.[75] The JHR is a therapeutic shock reaction that occurs within 24 hours of the start of therapy and is associated with a dramatic worsening of clinical symptoms in approximately 5% of cases. This reaction is believed to occur through a pronounced release of pyrogenic cytokines with significant elevation in the levels of tumor necrosis factor (TNF)-α, IL-6, and IL-8.[76] Some have reported benefit from use of anti-TNF-α.[77] Although some studies have documented use of single-dose therapeutic regimes, more commonly antimicrobials are given for 7 to 14 days. **Table 2** details some of the more commonly used treatment dosages and regimens.[78]

Mortality rates vary with the infecting agent, with most TBRF cases having less than 5% mortality. Mortality can be higher, however, with the East African species *B duttonii* and its louse-borne variant, *B recurrentis*. Particularly high perinatal mortality rates reaching 475 cases per 1000 pregnant women have been reported from Tanzania where *B duttonii* is endemic. Higher spirochetal loads are reported among pregnant individuals compared with nonpregnant controls.[79] Life-long protection postinfection

Table 2
Treatment options commonly used for relapsing fever management

Antibiotic	Dosage Used	Duration	Comments
Penicillin	400,000–600,000 IU daily	7–14 d	Single dose can be curative for LBRF CNS involvement
Tetracycline	200–250 mg bid to 500 mg qid	7–14 d	Single dose can be curative for LBRF
Doxycycline	200–250 mg (4 mg/kg/d)	7–14 d	Prophylaxis (200 mg day 1, then 100 mg daily 4 d postexposure) or for treatment
Erythromycin	2 g daily (50 mg/kg children)	7–14 d	Pregnancy or children
Chloramphenicol	500 mg 6 hourly (12.5 mg/kg children)	7–14 d	Pregnancy or children
Ceftriaxone	2 g daily	7–14 d	CNS involvement

Abbreviation: CNS, central nervous system.

does not seem to be the norm, with repeat infections being reported among individuals residing in endemic regions.

DIAGNOSTIC METHODS
Microscopy

Although refractory to visualization by Gram staining, these spirochetes can be stained using Giemsa stain, Wright stain, or silver staining methods (**Fig. 7**). Darkfield or phase microscopy can be used for freshly collected blood or cerebrospinal fluid if available (or to check results of cultivation or after animal inoculation), enabling observation of the highly motile spirochetes. Assessment of ticks for infection has used salivary glands, hemolymph extracted after leg amputation, or whole tick preparations. Although these methods can detect *Borrelia*, sensitivity is poor, requiring in excess of 10^5 organisms per milliliter for detection, particularly challenging for some species such as *B crocidurae*, for which the blood burden is lower than that of, for example, *B recurrentis*. Use of thick blood films can improve sensitivity if numbers are low, but alternative methods such as molecular detection might provide more reliable data if sensitivity is a priority. This method is further complicated by the need to collect blood during febrile episodes. An additional limitation of direct microscopy is the inability to differentiate the causative species.

Animal Inoculation

Animal inoculation, particularly use of small rodents, was popular both for its ability to recover cultivable strains[80] and to identify these agents through comparative virulence studies (mice and guinea pigs).[8] Although now not routinely undertaken, this technique is largely restricted to specialist institutes where it remains useful for recovery of

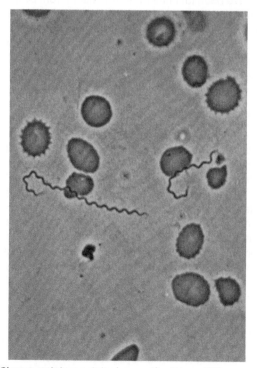

Fig. 7. Blood film (Giemsa staining; original magnification ×400).

primary isolates. On a cautionary note, some species, such as *B recurrentis*, are refractory to growth in rodent models but can be isolated in primate models. Use of immunocompromised SCID mice to overcome this limitation was met with mixed success, with only low-level infection being achieved.[81]

Cultivation

Isolation of relapsing fever borreliae can also be achieved in culture by directly inoculating clinical samples into specialized liquid media (such as Barbour-Stoenner-Kelly (BSKII) or Modified Kelly-Pettenkofer [MKP]). However, the fastidious, slow-growing nature of these spirochetes makes this technically demanding.[82–84] Not all batches of commercially produced medium support growth equally well, and consequently, batch testing of media should be used. In cases of culture contamination, inclusion of antimicrobials such as rifampicin, colistin sulfate, aminoglycosides, or antifungals can be used to help purify isolates. Alternatively, the slender *Borrelia* morphology enables purification of contaminated cultures through filtration.

Not all species or strains are uniformly cultivable.[12] Until the 1990s, *B recurrentis* and *B duttonii* were deemed noncultivable until isolates were successfully recovered using BSKII medium.[85–87] Despite the successful isolation of *B duttonii*, comparison of genotypes recovered by cultivation and those detected by polymerase chain reaction/sequencing directly from ticks revealed that all cultivable isolates belonged to only 1 of the 4 genotypic groups prevalent in the study area.[12]

Serologic Detection

Specific antigens, including GlpQ and BipA, that are shared by all relapsing fever group spirochetes have been identified but are absent from *Borrelia* species associated with Lyme disease, thus precluding serologic cross-reactions between these borreliae.[88,89] These antigens have been used successfully in enzyme-linked immunoassays to enable serologic diagnosis or population screening. However, such assays have not been produced commercially, as they would have little value in highly endemic regions and the sporadic nature of imported cases makes commercialization financially nonviable.

Molecular Detection

Molecular detection and identification approaches offer distinct advantages over the recovery of these fastidious microbes and has become the mainstay for both detection and typing of relapsing fever *Borrelia*. Various conserved targets, such as 16S rRNA and flagellin (*flaB*) genes, have been used for diagnosis but lack discriminatory power for typing.[34,90,91] Availability of genomic sequence data has enabled development of single nucleotide polymorphism–based multiplex identification methods and highly discriminatory multispacer typing methods.[92,93] It must be remembered that these assays may not always detect newly described species. Use of 16S-23S ribosomal intragenic spacer region sequencing has provided a highly discriminatory means of delineating strains.[12] Application of these high-resolution methods has enabled scrutiny of the genotypes circulating in specific enzootic regions and correlation with tick and vertebrate species.[4]

Proteomics

Although the application of proteomics for detection of relapsing fever borreliosis is in its infancy, this is an exciting potential application. Differences in proteomic profiles have been detected, differentiating tick hemolymph derived from *Borrelia*-infected ticks and their uninfected counterparts. This method could provide a more cost-effective means of screening ticks for carriage of relapsing fever spirochetes.[94]

CONTROL AND INTERVENTION

Relapsing fever spirochetes are exquisitely susceptible to antimicrobials including penicillin, tetracycline/doxycycline, chloramphenicol, ceftriaxone, and erythromycin. Wide use of antimicrobials coupled with improvements in living conditions, particularly in areas where relapsing fever has its reservoir in humans, such as LBRF in Ethiopia, has been correlated with a declining incidence of infection.[62]

This decline is not so apparent for the tick-borne forms of the disease that persist in their longer-lived tick vector/reservoirs and through the zoonotic vertebrate reservoirs. The burden of TBRF among subsistence agropastoralist communities in developing nations remains substantial. Use of acaracides (including arsenicals, chlorinated hydrocarbons, organophosphates, carbamates, and synthetic pyrethroids) has been met with some success, although costs are prohibitive in many areas that would benefit from use of such measures, and the environmental consequences of their use should not be overlooked.[95,96] Biological controls have been explored, with entomopathogenic fungi showing some success against ixodid ticks, but control of argasid ticks has been largely neglected.[97–99]

Prohibiting access to high-risk areas has successfully reduced disease incidence in areas endemic for *Borrelia persica* in Israel where significant levels of infection occurred among military personnel while using tick-infested caves during training. If contact is unavoidable, doxycycline prophylaxis has been used for short-term prevention.[100]

Given the limitations of acaricides to reduce the burden of infection, other options such as immunologic controls have also been explored. These measures have been used to reduce relapsing fever and other pathogens vectored by the same tick species, such as African swine fever virus, a hemorrhagic febrile infection of swine with a mortality rate approaching 100%. Control at the level of the vector is consequently an attractive prospect. Again, anti-tick vaccines against ixodid ticks have led the way, with commercial vaccines against *Rhipicephalus microplus* being marketed in Australia and Latin America.[96] Analysis of both the gut transcriptome and proteome of argasid ticks is an essential prerequisite for the development of such vaccine candidates. Whether these potential vaccines would be directed primarily toward protection of livestock or companion animals from tick-borne infection, or whether a one health approach, whereby reduction of ticks through protection of their vertebrate hosts would indirectly reduce human infections, remains to be resolved.

CONCLUDING REMARKS

The relapsing fever *Borrelia* have a long and notorious history, from being one of the earliest bacterial infectious diseases described associated with high mortality and morbidity through to a period of neglect. This neglect in part was a result of the demise of the clothing louse and hence also LBRF, through improved hygiene and living conditions and use of dichlorodiphenyltrichloroethane. Similarly, improvements in housing have reduced contact between soft ticks and humans, except in areas of poverty. Despite these global reductions in relapsing fever, endemic regions persist and detection of cases is often suboptimal. Clinical overlap with malaria and use of suboptimal diagnostic methods for relapsing fever agents hamper the detection of this treatable infection.

Despite this neglect, application of improved methods for detection, typing, and cultivation of these spirochetes has allowed us to gain intriguing insights into the biology of these organisms. Newly described species and deeper understanding of the previously established members of this group will help us dissect evolutionary and ecological relationships. Greater insights into the mechanisms of pathogenesis and strategies used to evade the immune defenses of the vertebrate host will provide future research goals.

SELF-ASSESSMENT

1. What is the time required for argasid ticks to feed to repletion?
   a. 5 minutes to 2 hours
   b. Greater than 48 hours
   c. 1 to 10 seconds
   d. Greater than 7 days
2. Which of the following statements regarding relapsing fever borreliosis is incorrect?
   a. These infections are acquired from arthropods, including lice and ticks.
   b. This infection is a strictly tropical disease.
   c. Reinfection can occur.
   d. Infection can be treated with antibiotics such as penicillin or doxycycline.
3. Which of the following relapsing fever borreliae are not considered to be zoonotic?
   a. *Borrelia persica* and *Borrelia microti*
   b. *Borrelia crocidurae* and *Borrelia hispanica*
   c. *Borrelia hermsii* and *Borrelia turicatae*
   d. *Borrelia recurrentis* and *Borrelia duttonii*
4. *Borrelia recurrentis* is believed to have evolved from which of the tick-borne relapsing fever borreliae?
   a. *Borrelia hermsii*
   b. *Borrelia duttonii*
   c. *Borrelia persica*
   d. *Borrelia hispanica*
5. Which vertebrate species is believed to have an important role in the ecology of relapsing fever in California?
   a. Flying squirrel
   b. Rat
   c. Bats
   d. Chipmunk

Answers
   Answer 1: A
   Answer 2: B
   Answer 3: D
   Answer 4: B
   Answer 5: D

REFERENCES

1. Birkhaug K, Otto HF. Obermeier. In: Moulton FR, editor. A symposium on relapsing fever in the Americas. Washington, DC: American Association for the Advancement of Science. Section on Medical Sciences; 1942. p. 7–9.
2. Bryceson ADM, Parry EHO, Perine PL, et al. Louse-borne relapsing fever: a clinical and laboratory study of 62 cases in Ethiopia and a reconsideration of the literature. Q J Med 1970;39:129–70.

3. Cutler SJ, Abdissa A, Trape JF. New concepts for the old challenge of African relapsing fever borreliosis. Clin Microbiol Infect 2009;15:400–6.

4. Schwan TG, Anderson JM, Lopez JE, et al. Endemic foci of the tick-borne relapsing fever spirochete Borrelia crocidurae in Mali, West Africa, and the potential for human infection. PLoS Negl Trop Dis 2012;6(11):e1924.

5. Ross PH, Milne AD. Tick fever. Br Med J 1904;ii:1453–4.

6. Dutton JE, Todd JL. The nature of tick fever in the eastern part of the Congo Free State. Br Med J 1905;ii:1259–60.

7. Mitani H, Talbert A, Fukunaga M. New World relapsing fever Borrelia found in Ornithodoros porcinus ticks in central Tanzania. Microbiol Immunol 2004;48: 501–5.

8. Naddaf SR, Ghazinezhad B, Bahramali G, et al. Phylogenetic analysis of the spirochete Borrelia microti, a potential agent of relapsing fever in Iran. J Clin Microbiol 2012;50:2873–6.

9. Naddaf S, Ghazinezhad B, Sedaghat M, et al. Tickborne relapsing fever in southern Iran, 2011–2013. Emerg Infect Dis 2015;21:1078–80.

10. Schwan TG, Raffel SJ, Schrumpf ME, et al. Characterization of a novel relapsing fever spirochete in the midgut, coxal fluid, and salivary glands of the bat tick Carios kelleyi. Vector Borne Zoonotic Dis 2009;9:643–7.

11. Yabsley MJ, Parsons NJ, Horne EC, et al. Novel relapsing fever Borrelia detected in African penguins (Spheniscus demersus) admitted to two rehabilitation centers in South Africa. Parasitol Res 2012;110:1125–30.

12. Cutler SJ, Margarita Bonilla E, Singh RJ. Population structure of East African relapsing fever Borrelia spp. Emerg Infect Dis 2010;16:1076–80.

13. Ras NM, Lascola B, Postic D, et al. Phylogenesis of relapsing fever Borrelia spp. Int J Syst Bacteriol 1996;46:859–65.

14. Lescot M, Audic S, Robert C, et al. The genome of Borrelia recurrentis, the agent of deadly louse-borne relapsing fever, is a degraded subset of tick-borne Borrelia duttonii. PLoS Genet 2008;4(9):e1000185.

15. Elbir H, Gimenez G, Robert C, et al. Complete genome sequence of Borrelia crocidurae. J Bacteriol 2012;194:3723–4.

16. Barbour AG, Hayes SF. Biology of Borrelia species. Microbiol Rev 1986;50: 381–400.

17. Bárcena-Uribarri I, Thein M, Sacher A, et al. P66 porins are present in both Lyme disease and relapsing fever spirochetes: a comparison of the biophysical properties of P66 porins from six Borrelia species. Biochim Biophys Acta 2010;1798: 1197–203.

18. Thein M, Bunikis I, Denker K, et al. Oms38 is the first identified pore-forming protein in the outer membrane of relapsing fever spirochetes. J Bacteriol 2008;190: 7035–42.

19. Thein M, Bonde M, Bunikis I, et al. DipA, a pore-forming protein in the outer membrane of Lyme disease spirochetes exhibits specificity for the permeation of dicarboxylates. PLoS One 2012;7(5):e36523.

20. Magoun L, Zückert WR, Robbins D, et al. Variable small protein (Vsp)-dependent and Vsp-independent pathways for glycosaminoglycan recognition by relapsing fever spirochaetes. Mol Microbiol 2000;36:886–97.

21. Londoño D, Cadavid D. Bacterial lipoproteins can disseminate from the periphery to inflame the brain. Am J Pathol 2010;176:2848–57.

22. Guo BP, Teneberg S, Munch R, et al. Relapsing fever Borrelia binds to neolacto glycans and mediates rosetting of human erythrocytes. Proc Natl Acad Sci U S A 2009;106:19280–5.

23. Shamaei-Tousi A, Martin P, Bergh A, et al. Erythrocyte-aggregating relapsing fever spirochete *Borrelia crocidurae* induces formation of microemboli. J Infect Dis 1999;180:1929–38.

24. Miller SC, Porcella SF, Raffel SJ, et al. Large linear plasmids of *Borrelia* species that cause relapsing fever. J Bacteriol 2013;195:3629–39.

25. Restrepo BI, Kitten T, Carter CJ, et al. Subtelomeric expression regions of *Borrelia hermsii* linear plasmids are highly polymorphic. Mol Microbiol 1992;6: 3299–311.

26. Di L, Pagan PE, Packer D, et al. BorreliaBase: a phylogeny-centered browser of *Borrelia* genomes. BMC Bioinformatics 2014;15:233.

27. Socolovschi C, Kernif T, Raoult D, et al. *Borrelia*, *Rickettsia*, and *Ehrlichia* species in bat ticks, France, 2010. Emerg Infect Dis 2012;18:1966–75.

28. Loftis A, Gill J, Schriefer M, et al. Detection of *Rickettsia*, *Borrelia*, and *Bartonella* in *Carios kelleyi* (Acari: argasidae). J Med Entomol 2005;42:473–80.

29. Reeves W, Loftis A, Sanders F, et al. *Borrelia*, *Coxiella*, and *Rickettsia* in *Carios capensis* (Acari: Argasidae) from a brown pelican (*Pelecanus occidentalis*) rookery in South Carolina, USA. Exp Appl Acarol 2006;39:321–9.

30. Takano A, Sugimori C, Fujita H, et al. A novel relapsing fever *Borrelia* sp. infects the salivary glands of the molted hard tick, *Amblyomma geoemydae*. Ticks Tick Borne Dis 2012;3:259–61.

31. McCoy BN, Maïga O, Schwan TG. Detection of *Borrelia theileri* in *Rhipicephalus geigyi* from Mali. Ticks Tick Borne Dis 2014;5:401–3.

32. Cutler S, Abdissa A, Adamu H, et al. Borrelia in Ethiopian ticks. Ticks Tick Borne Dis 2012;3:14–7.

33. Yparraguirre LA, Machado-Ferreira E, Ullmann AJ, et al. A hard tick relapsing fever group spirochete in a Brazilian *Rhipicephalus* (*Boophilus*) *microplus*. Vector Borne Zoonotic Dis 2007;7:717–21.

34. Kumsa B, Socolovschi C, Raoult D, et al. New *Borrelia* species detected in ixodid ticks in Oromia, Ethiopia. Ticks Tick Borne Dis 2015;6:401–7.

35. Mediannikov O, Abdissa A, Socolovschi C, et al. Detection of a new *Borrelia* species in ticks taken from cattle in southwest Ethiopia. Vector Borne Zoonotic Dis 2013;13:266–9.

36. Lane RS, Mun J, Parker JM, et al. Columbian black-tailed deer (*Odocoileus hemionus columbianus*) as hosts for *Borrelia* spp. in northern California. J Wildl Dis 2005;41:115–25.

37. Thomas NJ, Bunikis J, Barbour AG, et al. Fatal spirochetosis due to a relapsing fever-like *Borrelia* sp. in a northern spotted owl. J Wildl Dis 2002;38:187–93.

38. Evans N, Bown K, Timofte D, et al. Fatal borreliosis in bat caused by relapsing fever spirochete, United Kingdom. Emerg Infect Dis 2009;15:1331.

39. Trape JF. Morbidity record in Africa for an unrecognized emergent disease. Cahiers Sante 2006;16:102.

40. Brouqui P, Stein A, Dupont H, et al. Ectoparasitism and vector-borne diseases in 930 homeless people from Marseilles. Medicine (Baltimore) 2005;84:61–8.

41. Li W, Ortiz G, Fournier P-E, et al. Genotyping of human lice suggests multiple emergences of body lice from local head louse populations. PLoS Negl Trop Dis 2010;4:e641.

42. Light JE, Allen JM, Long LM, et al. Geographic distributions and origins of human head lice (*Pediculus humanus* capitis) based on mitochondrial data. J Parasitol 2008;94:1275–81.

43. Boutellis A, Mediannikov O, Bilcha KD, et al. *Borrelia recurrentis* in head lice, Ethiopia. Emerg Infect Dis 2013;19:796–8.

44. Angelakis E, Rolain JM, Raoult D, et al. *Bartonella quintana* in head louse nits. FEMS Immunol Med Microbiol 2011;62:244–6.
45. Boutellis A, Veracx A, Angelakis E, et al. *Bartonella quintana* in head lice from Sénégal. Vector Borne Zoonotic Dis 2012;12:564–7.
46. Cutler S, Abdissa A, Adamu H, et al. *Bartonella quintana* in Ethiopian lice. Comp Immunol Microbiol Infect Dis 2012;35:17–21.
47. Moran-Gilad J, Levine H, Schwartz E, et al. Postexposure prophylaxis of tick-borne relapsing fever: lessons learned from recent outbreaks in Israel. Vector Borne Zoonotic Dis 2013;13:791–7.
48. Colebunders R, De Serrano P, Van Gompel A, et al. Imported relapsing fever in European tourists. Scand J Infect Dis 1993;25:533–6.
49. Wyplosz B, Mihaila-Amrouche L, Baixench M-T, et al. Imported tickborne relapsing fever, France. Emerg Infect Dis 2005;11:1801–3.
50. Rummens JL, Louwagie A, Van Hoof A, et al. Relapsing fever imported into Belgium: a case report. Acta Clin Belg 1987;42:210–4.
51. Kutsuna S, Kawabata H, Kasahara K, et al. Case report: the first case of imported relapsing fever in Japan. Am J Trop Med Hyg 2013;89:460–1.
52. Schwan TG, Policastro PF, Miller Z, et al. Tick-borne relapsing fever caused by *Borrelia hermsii*, Montana. Emerg Infect Dis 2003;9:1151–4.
53. Trape JF, Godeluck B, Diatta G, et al. The spread of tick-borne borreliosis in West Africa and its relationship to sub-Saharan drought. Am J Trop Med Hyg 1996;54:289–93.
54. Cutler SJ. Relapsing fever - a forgotten disease revealed. J Appl Microbiol 2010; 108:1115–22.
55. Nordstrand A, Bunikis I, Larsson C, et al. Tickborne relapsing fever diagnosis obscured by malaria, Togo. Emerg Infect Dis 2007;13:117–23.
56. Diatta G, Souidi Y, Granjon L, et al. Epidemiology of tick-borne borreliosis in Morocco. PLoS Negl Trop Dis 2012;6(9):e1810.
57. Lundqvist J, Larsson C, Nelson M, et al. Concomitant infection decreases the malaria burden but escalates relapsing fever borreliosis. Infect Immun 2010; 78:1924–30.
58. Parola P, Diatta G, Socolovschi C, et al. Tick-borne relapsing fever borreliosis, rural Senegal. Emerg Infect Dis 2011;17:883–5.
59. Sarih M, Garnier M, Boudebouch N, et al. *Borrelia hispanica* relapsing fever, Morocco. Emerg Infect Dis 2009;15:1626–9.
60. Schwan TG, Raffel SJ, Schrumpf ME, et al. Tick-borne relapsing fever and *Borrelia hermsii*, Los Angeles County, California, USA. Emerg Infect Dis 2009;15: 1026–31.
61. Trevejo RT, Schriefer ME, Gage KL, et al. An interstate outbreak of tick-borne relapsing fever among vacationers at a Rocky Mountain cabin. Am J Trop Med Hyg 1998;58:743–7.
62. Ramos JM, Malmierca E, Reyes F, et al. Results of a 10-year survey of louse-borne relapsing fever in southern Ethiopia: a decline in endemicity. Ann Trop Med Parasitol 2008;102:467–9.
63. Cadavid D, Londoño D. Understanding tropism and immunopathological mechanisms of relapsing fever spirochaetes. Clin Microbiol Infect 2009;15: 415–21.
64. Cadavid D, Sondey M, Garcia E, et al. Residual brain infection in relapsing-fever borreliosis. J Infect Dis 2006;193:1451–8.
65. Mehra R, Londoño D, Sondey M, et al. Structure-function investigation of Vsp serotypes of the spirochete *Borrelia hermsii*. PLoS One 2009;4(10):e7597.

66. Cadavid D, Pennington PM, Kerentseva TA, et al. Immunologic and genetic analyses of VmpA of a neurotropic strain of *Borrelia turicatae*. Infect Immun 1997; 65:3352–60.
67. Sethi N, Sondey M, Bai Y, et al. Interaction of a neurotropic strain of *Borrelia turicatae* with the cerebral microcirculation system. Infect Immun 2006;74: 6408–18.
68. Larsson C, Andersson M, Pelkonen J, et al. Persistent brain infection and disease reactivation in relapsing fever borreliosis. Microbes Infect 2006;8: 2213–9.
69. Dai Q, Restrepo BI, Porcella SF, et al. Antigenic variation by *Borrelia hermsii* occurs through recombination between extragenic repetitive elements on linear plasmids. Mol Microbiol 2006;60:1329–43.
70. Rossmann E, Kraiczy P, Herzberger P, et al. BhCRASP-1 of the relapsing fever spirochete *Borrelia hermsii* is a factor H- and plasminogen-binding protein. Int J Med Microbiol 2008;298:272–83.
71. Grosskinsky S, Schott M, Brenner C, et al. *Borrelia recurrentis* employs a novel multifunctional surface protein with anti-complement, anti-opsonic and invasive potential to escape innate immunity. PLoS One 2009;4(3):e4858.
72. Borgnolo G, Hailu B, Ciancarelli A, et al. Louse-borne relapsing fever. A clinical and an epidemiological study of 389 patients in Asella Hospital, Ethiopia. Trop Geogr Med 1993;45:66–9.
73. Borgnolo G, Denku B, Chiabrera F, et al. Louse-borne relapsing fever in Ethiopian children: a clinical study. Ann Trop Paediatr 1993;13:165–71.
74. Brown V, Larouze B, Desve G, et al. Clinical presentation of louse-born relapsing fever among Ethiopian refugees in northern Somalia. Ann Trop Med Parasitol 1988;82:499–502.
75. Guerrier G, Doherty T. Comparison of antibiotic regimens for treating louse-borne relapsing fever: a meta-analysis. Trans R Soc Trop Med Hyg 2011;105: 483–90.
76. Negussie Y, Remick DG, DeForge LE, et al. Detection of plasma tumor necrosis factor, interleukins 6, and 8 during the Jarisch-Herxheimer reaction of relapsing fever. J Exp Med 1992;175:1207–12.
77. Fekade D, Knox K, Hussein K, et al. Prevention of Jarisch-Herxheimer reactions by treatment with antibodies against tumor necrosis factor α. N Engl J Med 1996;335:311–5.
78. Belum GR, Belum VR, Chaitanya Arudra SK, et al. The Jarisch–Herxheimer reaction: revisited. Travel Med Infect Dis 2013;11(4):231–7.
79. Jongen VH, van Roosmalen J, Tiems J, et al. Tick-borne relapsing fever and pregnancy outcome in rural Tanzania. Acta Obstet Gynecol Scand 1997;76: 834–8.
80. Fritz CL, Bronson LR, Smith CR, et al. Isolation and characterization of *Borrelia hermsii* associated with two foci of tick-borne relapsing fever in California. J Clin Microbiol 2004;42:1123–8.
81. Larsson C, Lundqvist J, van Rooijen N, et al. A novel animal model of *Borrelia recurrentis* louse-borne relapsing fever borreliosis using immunodeficient mice. PLoS Negl Trop Dis 2009;3:e522.
82. Barbour A. Isolation and cultivation of Lyme disease spirochetes. Yale J Biol Med 1984;57:521–5.
83. Wagemakers A, Oei A, Fikrig MM, et al. The relapsing fever spirochete *Borrelia miyamotoi* is cultivable in a modified Kelly-Pettenkofer medium, and is resistant to human complement. Parasit Vectors 2014;7:418.

84. Cutler SJ, Jones SE, Wright DJM, et al. Cultivation of East African relapsing fever *Borrelia* and review of preceding events. J Spirochetal Tick Borne Dis 2000;7: 52–8.

85. Cutler SJ, Akintunde COK, Moss J, et al. Successful in vitro cultivation of *Borrelia duttonii* and its comparison with *Borrelia recurrentis*. Int J Syst Bacteriol 1999;49: 1793–9.

86. Cutler S, Moss J, Fukunaga M, et al. *Borrelia recurrentis* characterization and comparison with relapsing fever, Lyme-associated, and other *Borrelia* spp. Int J Syst Bacteriol 1997;47:958–68.

87. Cutler SJ, Fekade D, Hussein K, et al. Successful in-vitro cultivation of *Borrelia recurrentis*. Lancet 1994;343:242.

88. Schwan TG, Schrumpf ME, Hinnebusch BJ, et al. GlpQ: an antigen for serological discrimination between relapsing fever and Lyme borreliosis. J Clin Microbiol 1996;34:2483–92.

89. Lopez J, Schrumpf M, Nagarajan V, et al. A novel surface antigen of relapsing fever spirochetes can discriminate between relapsing fever and Lyme borreliosis. Clin Vaccine Immunol 2010;17:564–71.

90. Fukunaga M, Ushijima Y, Aoki L, et al. Detection of *Borrelia duttoni*, a tick-borne relapsing fever agent in central Tanzania, within ticks by flagellin gene-based nested polymerase chain reaction. Vector Borne Zoonotic Dis 2001;1:331–8.

91. Assous MV, Wilamowski A, Bercovier H, et al. Molecular characterization of tick-borne relapsing fever *Borrelia*, Israel. Emerg Infect Dis 2006;12:1740–3.

92. Elbir H, Henry M, Diatta G, et al. Multiplex real-time PCR diagnostic of relapsing fevers in Africa. PLoS Negl Trop Dis 2013;7(1):e2042.

93. Elbir H, Gimenez G, Sokhna C, et al. Multispacer sequence typing relapsing fever borreliae in Africa. PLoS Negl Trop Dis 2012;6(6):e1652.

94. Fotso Fotso A, Mediannikov O, Diatta G, et al. MALDI-TOF mass spectrometry detection of pathogens in vectors: the *Borrelia crocidurae/Ornithodoros sonrai* paradigm. PLoS Negl Trop Dis 2014;8:e2984.

95. Talbert A, Nyange A, Molteni F. Spraying tick-infested houses with lambda-cyhalothrin reduces the incidence of tick-borne relapsing fever in children under five years old. Trans R Soc Trop Med Hyg 1998;92:251–3.

96. Díaz-Martín V, Manzano-Román R, Obolo-Mvoulouga P, et al. Development of vaccines against *Ornithodoros* soft ticks: an update. Ticks Tick Borne Dis 2015;6:211–20.

97. D'Alessandro WB, Humber RA, Luz C. Occurrence of pathogenic fungi to *Amblyomma cajennense* in a rural area of Central Brazil and their activities against vectors of Rocky Mountain spotted fever. Vet Parasitol 2012;188:156–9.

98. Greengarten PJ, Tuininga AR, Morath SU, et al. Occurrence of soil- and tick-borne fungi and related virulence tests for pathogenicity to *Ixodes scapularis* (Acari: Ixodidae). J Med Entomol 2011;48:337–44.

99. Tavassoli M, Malekifard F, Soleimanzadeh A, et al. Susceptibility of different life stages of *Ornithodoros lahorensis* to entomopathogenic fungi *Metarhizium anisopliae* and *Beauveria bassiana*. Parasitol Res 2012;111:1779–83.

100. Assous MV, Wilamowski A. Relapsing fever borreliosis in Eurasia - forgotten, but certainly not gone! Clin Microbiol Infect 2009;15:407–14.

Borrelia miyamotoi Disease

Neither Lyme Disease Nor Relapsing Fever

Sam R. Telford III, ScD[a],*, Heidi K. Goethert, ScD[a], Philip J. Molloy, MD[b],
Victor P. Berardi[b], Hanumara Ram Chowdri, MD[c],
Joseph L. Gugliotta, MD[d], Timothy J. Lepore, MD[e]

KEYWORDS

- *Borrelia miyamotoi* • Lyme disease • Deer ticks • Borreliosis • Zoonotic infection

KEY POINTS

- *Borrelia miyamotoi* was first described from Japanese *Ixodes persulcatus* ticks. Subsequently, it was detected as an inherited infection of *Ixodes dammini* ticks in the northeastern United States.
- The index case of *B miyamotoi* disease (BMD) in the United States comprised meningoencephalitis in an elderly immunocompromised patient. BMD is likely a common, underdiagnosed zoonosis wherever Lyme disease is reported.
- Cases typically present with headache, fever, chills, fatigue, and myalgia. BMD should not be considered a relapsing fever; there is no crisis with rigors or hyperpyrexia followed by diaphoresis and hypotension.
- BMD may be confirmed by PCR of acute blood samples or by seroconversion to a recombinant GlpQ antigen.
- Treatment is identical to that for Lyme disease.

Potential Conflicts of Interest: V.P. Berardi is an associate director of laboratory science and CEO of Imugen, Inc. P.J. Molloy and H.K. Goethert are employees of Imugen, Inc. H.R. Chowdri is a clinical consultant and S.R. Telford is a consultant and scientific advisor to Imugen, Inc.
S.R. Telford and H.K. Goethert are supported, in part, by grants from the National Institutes of Health (U01AI109656, R41AI078631); the Tufts Innovation Institute; the Evelyn Lilly Lutz Foundation; the Dorothy Harrison Egan Foundation; and the Bill and Melinda Gates Foundation.
[a] Department of Infectious Disease and Global Health, Tufts University, Cummings School of Veterinary Medicine, 200 Westboro Road, North Grafton, MA 01536, USA; [b] Imugen, Inc., 315 Norwood Park South, Norwood, MA 02062, USA; [c] Hawthorn Medical Associates, 275 Allen Street, Unit 3, New Bedford, MA 02740, USA; [d] Hunterdon Medical Center Infectious Diseases, 1100 Wescott Drive, Suite 306, Flemington, NJ 08822, USA; [e] Nantucket Cottage Hospital, 57 Prospect Street, Nantucket, MA 02554, USA
* Corresponding author.
E-mail address: sam.telford@tufts.edu

INTRODUCTION

Tick borne *Borrelia* spp are now usually divided into two taxonomic groups, which correspond to the typical human disease manifestations, Lyme disease and relapsing fever, and to their tick vectors, prostriate ixodid ticks and argasid ticks, respectively (**Table 1**). Theiler[1] demonstrated spirochetes in metastriate ixodid ticks infesting African cattle with a mild disease that was called "tick spirochetosis" or bovine borreliosis. *Borrelia theileri* subsequently has been globally reported, usually associated with cattle and their cosmopolitan tick *Rhipicephalus (Boophilus) microplus* and *Rhipicephalus annulatus*. Professor Kenji Miyamoto of Asahikawa Medical College, during 1990 to 1992, isolated spirochetes from *Ixodes persulcatus* ticks collected in Hokkaido, Japan. These isolates were subsequently demonstrated by analysis of the 23S-5S rDNA and other genes to be a new species related to the relapsing fever spirochetes.[2] The name *Borrelia miyamotoi* was applied to this new species, and subsequently, this spirochete has been detected wherever *I persulcatus* species complex ticks (*Ixodes dammini*, *Ixodes scapularis*, *Ixodes pacificus*, *Ixodes ricinus*, herein referred to as *Ixodes* spp) occur. In 1995, borreliae from American Lone Star ticks (*Amblyomma americanum*) were identified independently by two research groups[3,4] and provided the names *Borrelia lonestari* and *Borrelia barbouri*; the former name has prevailed in the literature.[1] Molecular phylogenetic analyses demonstrate that *B theileri*, *B lonestari*, and *B miyamotoi* comprise a group together, deep within the relapsing fever spirochete clade[5] and not within the other ixodid ("hard") tick maintained borreliae, namely those in *Ixodes* spp that are recognized as *Borrelia burgdorferi* sensu lato. Although phylogenetically considered to be relapsing fever spirochetes, the metastriate-transmitted *Borrelia* spp should not be assumed to be biologically similar to the true relapsing fever spirochetes maintained by argasid ("soft") ticks, or to cause typical relapsing fever.

As with *B burgdorferi* (discussed elsewhere in this issue), evidence is emerging that *B miyamotoi* comprises a species complex or group of genospecies[5] and should be referred to as *B miyamotoi* sensu lato. Asian, European, and American clades are apparent with phylogenetic analyses of typical gene targets, such as flagellin (**Fig. 1**). Unlike *B burgdorferi* s.l., for which less than half of the recognized genospecies have been associated with human infection, all three *B miyamotoi* clades recognized thus far have been associated with human clinical cases.

The biology of *B theileri* has been well studied, particularly clinical aspects of bovine borreliosis[6] and vector-pathogen interactions.[7] *B lonestari* has been circumstantially associated with a disease manifesting mainly as erythema migrans (southern tick–associated rash illness, or Masters disease), but its formal incrimination as the etiologic agent remains lacking.[8] Further discussion of southern tick–associated rash illness/ Masters disease as a borreliosis is beyond the scope of this article. *B miyamotoi*, despite its global distribution in Lyme disease vectors, remained as an incidental finding in field surveys and was thought to be an endosymbiont of *Ixodes* spp ticks. In 2011, a case series comprising febrile Russian patients, some with a recurrent fever, was presented with polymerase chain reaction (PCR) evidence that implicated *B miyamotoi* as the etiologic agent.[9] This was the first suggestion that *B miyamotoi* was capable of causing human disease, and was followed in 2013 by the index case for

---

[1] The name *B lonestari* technically should be presented in quotation marks or referred to as Candidatus *Borrelia lonestari*, in as much as the requirements for naming a new bacterial taxon have not been fulfilled, in particular, formal publication in the *International Journal of Systematic and Evolutionary Microbiology* and its propagation in vitro that would enable deposition of cultures into an accepted biologic repository.

Table 1
Kinds of ticks and their roles as vectors of *Borrelia* spp

Family	Subfamily	Colloquial Name	Species Example	Common Name	Associated *Borrelia* sp
Argasidae	Argasinae	Soft ticks	*Ornithodoros moubata*	Tampan tick	*B duttoni*
Ixodidae	(Division Prostriata)—Ixodinae	Hard ticks	*Ixodes persulcatus*	Taiga tick	*B burgdorferi* s.l., *B miyamotoi* s.l.
Ixodidae	(Division Metastriata)—Rhipicephalinae, Amblyomminae, Haemaphysalinae, Hyalomminae	Hard ticks	*Amblyomma americanum*	Lone Star tick	*B lonestari*

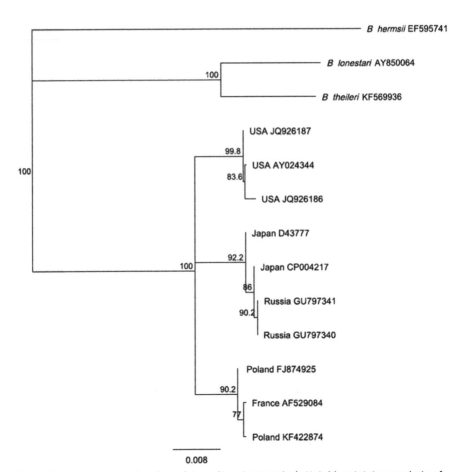

Fig. 1. Phylogenetic relationship of *Borrelia miyamotoi* s.l. Neighbor-joining analysis of a 608-bp portion of the flagellin gene. Numbers at nodes represent proportion of 1000 bootstrap replicates consistent with the branching topology; branch lengths are proportional to nucleotide differences. Three *B miyamotoi* clades are apparent: American, Japanese/Russian, and European. (*Data from* GenBank. Available at: http://www.ncbi.nlm.nih.gov/genbank/. Accessed May 8, 2015.)

North America[10] and soon thereafter that for the European Union.[11] It is now known that at least in the northeastern United States, *B miyamotoi* disease (BMD) may be relatively common.[12]

EPIDEMIOLOGY

BMD seems to be a common infection in sites that are intensely zoonotic for Lyme disease. For the Russian case series, BMD was diagnosed as frequently as tick-borne encephalitis and about half as frequently as erythema migrans caused by *B burgdorferi* s.l.[9] Active case detection using PCR of acute phase blood samples from 11,515 febrile patients in southern New England demonstrated that 3.1% had evidence of infection by *Babesia microti*, 1.4% by *Anaplasma phagocytophilum*, and 0.8% by *B miyamotoi*.[12] It should be noted that blood was sampled only from patients whose signs and symptoms were sufficient to cause them to seek medical attention; it is likely that subclinical *B miyamotoi* infections occur. Indeed, an enzyme immunoassay (EIA) using the recombinant *B miy*amotoi antigen glycerophosphodiester phosphodies-terase (rGlpQ), suggested that the serum of about 4% of participants from cross-sectional serosurveys in New England Lyme disease endemic sites was reactive; about 9% of these sera reacted to antigens of *B burgdorferi*.[13]

The Russian case series presented from May to August,[9] and had an estimated 12- to 16-day incubation period. Adult *I persulcatus*, the Lyme disease and tick-borne encephalitis vector in the Yekaterinburg area, seek hosts during May and June,[14] with nymphs and larvae appearing during June and activity extending into August. It is thus not clear which *I persulcatus* developmental stage transmits *B miyamotoi* to people in Russia. In southern New England, about 70% of all the BMD cases were diagnosed during July and August,[12] which incriminates larval *I dammini* as the main BMD vector because nymphal *I dammini* have their main period of activity during May to mid-July. Two-thirds of all Lyme disease cases in the northeastern United States are reported during June and July,[15] which demonstrates that nymphal *I dammini* are the main vector stage. Accordingly, BMD in the northeastern United States has a different epidemiologic pattern than does Lyme disease. Education about preventing Lyme disease typically focuses on temporal risk during early summer (June) and with the emergence of adult deer ticks during the fall (October–November). Larval deer ticks would be found in the same habitats as nymphs or adults, but would require more intimate contact with the ground and leaf litter for a person to become infested. As with Lyme disease, nymphal and adult *Ixodes* spp may transmit infection, with prevalence rates of *B miyamotoi* infection typically ranging from 1% to 10%.[16–19] However, for most tick-borne infections, an infected tick is a necessary but insufficient condition for risk: risk is instead determined by whether a tick is allowed to feed for an extended duration. Adult *Ixodes* spp tend to seek hosts during the colder months when people are dressed in a manner that inhibits tick attachment. Adults are also much bigger and more easily detected and removed. Nymphal *Ixodes* spp are empirically efficient vectors for Lyme disease, and the finding that more BMD cases coincide with the larval tick season of activity in the northeastern United States suggests that nymphs may not transmit *B miyamotoi* as efficiently as do larvae.

As with *B burgdorferi* s.l., diverse kinds of warm-blooded animals may serve as amplifying hosts for *B miyamotoi*. *B miyamotoi* is easily propagated in the laboratory in sigmondontine and murine rodents.[16] A common reservoir host for *B burgdorferi* in the eastern United States, the white-footed mouse (*Peromyscus leucopus*), is naturally infected by *B miyamotoi*.[20] European and Japanese rodents known to maintain *B burgdorferi* s.l. are also competent hosts for *B miyamotoi*.[21,22] *B miyamotoi* has been detected in blood or in ticks removed from passerine or galliform birds[23] and from ticks attached to deer (although it is not clear whether the tick was infected before infesting the deer or acquired infection from the deer). Whether specific vertebrate reservoirs are required for *B miyamotoi* perpetuation is not axiomatic.

TRANSMISSION

B miyamotoi was first isolated from host-seeking, unfed adult *I persulcatus* ticks,[2] which implied that spirochetes had been maintained through the molt from fed nymph to adult stage ticks (ie, transstadial transmission). The comprehensive report that established the endemicity of *B miyamotoi* in North America[16] confirmed transstadial transmission and by inheritance (ie, transovarial transmission). *B burgdorferi* s.l., in contrast, is inefficiently inherited, if at all,[24] whereas the classic relapsing fever spirochetes (eg, *Borrelia hermsi*, *Borrelia turicata*, *Borrelia crocidurae*, *Borrelia duttoni*) can be readily maintained by this mode of transmission, at least for as many as five generations.[25] Vertebrate hosts can serve to increase the prevalence of infection in the general tick population, and may even be required to maintain full pathogenicity. However, they may not be necessary for spirochetal persistence from generation to generation. The agent of bovine borreliosis, B theileri, is also maintained in this manner, although the hard ticks that transmit B theileri, Rhipicephalus microplus, are "one host" ticks that (unlike most ticks that detach after each bloodmeal) attach as larvae, feed, and quickly develop into nymphs and then adults in situ without leaving the individual host. B lonestari is found in host-seeking larval A americanum (Telford, unpublished data, 2001) and is likely to have inheritance as an important mode of perpetuation. Thus, the metastriate hard tick borreliae (B theileri, B lonestari, and B miyamotoi) shares aspects of the biology of the soft tick–transmitted relapsing fever spirochetes.

Although B burgdorferi s.l. requires reactivation within the feeding Ixodes spp before attaining infectivity, the true relapsing fever spirochetes apparently do not; isolates are readily made by homogenizing and injecting infected soft ticks into mice. Reactivation was first described for Rickettsia rickettsii, the agent of Rocky Mountain spotted fever.[26] Host-seeking wood ticks, Dermacentor andersoni, collected from zoonotic sites failed to induce productive infection in guinea pigs when homogenized and intraperitoneally injected, but those that were allowed to prefeed for 24 hours on uninfected animals, then homogenized and injected into uninfected guinea pigs induced a typical fatal infection. Heating ticks to 37°C for several hours also induced the activation of the dormant rickettsiae, as demonstrated by their capacity to cause lethal infection. Subsequently, virtually all hard tick–transmitted pathogens were recognized to require a similar reactivation to attain infectivity.[27] The molecular basis of reactivation has been elegantly studied in B burgdorferi s.l.[28] and is the reason for the minimum 24-hour delay between tick attachment and delivery of an infectious dose to initiate Lyme disease. Reactivation does not seem to occur with the soft tick–transmitted relapsing fever spirochetes, perhaps because soft ticks require only a few hours for feeding, in contrast to hard ticks, which require days. It is not known whether B miyamotoi requires reactivation during transmission by Ixodes spp. Accordingly, it is not clear whether prompt removal of feeding ticks may reduce the risk of acquiring BMD, as it does Lyme disease, although prompt removal might influence the quantum of infection (dose) delivered.

Because B miyamotoi causes spirochetemia and can be detected by PCR in acute blood samples of febrile individuals, it is possible that transfusion-transmitted cases will be described. Further supporting this possibility is the finding that infected mouse blood retains infectivity by syringe passage under storage conditions that are similar to those used in blood banking.[29] However, the capacity of B miyamotoi to persist in people who have recovered from acute illness remains unknown.

CLINICAL PRESENTATION

The BMD index cases in North America[10] and in the European Union[11] presented with meningoencephalitis. Both patients were elderly and had recently undergone chemotherapy for malignancy. BMD in both of these individuals was progressive, comprising memory and cognitive deficits, and spirochetes were detected in cerebrospinal fluid samples, demonstrating active intrathecal infection. For both patients, acute disease was entirely resolved following antibiotic treatment. How frequently B miyamotoi breaches the blood-brain barrier of otherwise healthy individuals remains to be determined, although in our large case series no sign of meningeal irritation or encephalitis was observed.[12]

In the Russian case series described previously,[9] it was noted that BMD generally presented with more systemic signs and symptoms, particularly headache and fever, compared with Lyme disease. Virtually all patients presented with fever (axillary temperature >37.2°C), fatigue, and headache, a statistically significant difference from the presentation of patients with Lyme disease. The next most common signs and symptoms were myalgia, chills, nausea, and arthralgia, characterizing 30% to 60% of the patients. Similarly, a series of PCR-positive patients from New England[12] almost always demonstrated fever, chills, headache, myalgia, and fatigue. Referring physicians often noted that patients with BMD exhibited more significant symptoms than patients with Lyme disease. In fact, BMD can be misdiagnosed as ehrlichiosis caused by *A phagocytophilum* or Ehrlichia spp.[30] In both case series, rashes were observed for fewer than 10% of the patients.

Although recurrent fever has been reported from 10% of the Russian and American BMD cases, classical relapsing fever is a very different disease clinically and biologically. Relapsing fever has a sudden onset of two or more episodes of high fever (ie, >39°C), with an interfebrile period of a few days. The fevers end with half an hour of rigors, hyperpyrexia, and hypertension followed by hours of diaphoresis and hypotension. Often the patient is also delirious during this period. The spleen is enlarged and jaundice may be apparent in these patients.[31] In most respects, relapsing fever is a very severe, acute disease compared with either BMD or Lyme disease. With respect to pathobiology, relapsing fever spirochetes are characterized by their evasion of the host immune response by antigenic variation[32] with progressive replacement of dozens of variable membrane proteins. No evidence has been presented to suggest the phenomenon of antigenic variation by *B miyamotoi*. Accordingly, even though *B miyamotoi* is phylogenetically a relapsing fever spirochete, BMD should not be considered relapsing fever.

Presented next are three case vignettes, representing the spectrum of BMD that we have observed.

Case 1. Uncomplicated Borrelia miyamotoi Disease

In late November, an active 70-year-old woman from southeastern Massachusetts presented to an urgent care center with 2 days of fever to 38.9°C, shaking chills, rigors, and headache. She denied nausea, vomiting, diarrhea, or upper respiratory symptoms. A "big" tick had been imbedded in her flank 2 weeks prior. Her past medical history was significant for hypertension, hyperlipidemia, reflux disease, and osteopenia. Blood was drawn and she was advised to take nonsteroidal anti-inflammatory drugs, rest, and hydrate. Her complete blood cell count (CBC) was normal and a rapid influenza test was negative. PCR demonstrated *B miyamotoi* DNA in the blood sample and 5 days after the initial presentation, the patient reported symptomatic improvement with the use of nonsteroidal anti-inflammatory drugs without antimicrobials. Her body aches and chills resolved, and the patient was otherwise well, but she continued to complain of residual fatigue. Skin examination revealed residual erythema at the site of the tick bite but no other rashes. She was started on doxycycline, 100 mg twice daily, and a repeat blood sample taken at this time was negative for *B miyamotoi* or other deer tick-borne infections. She was re-evaluated in late December after completion of the doxycycline course and complained of residual fatigue. She was seen again in late January feeling much better with her fatigue resolving.

Case 2. Human Anaplasmosis or Borrelia miyamotoi Disease?

A healthy 57-year-old woman from southeastern Massachusetts became acutely ill in early August with fevers and chills, headache, and joint and muscle pain. Two days after onset, she went to the community hospital emergency room because of increasing lethargy, where she was found to be febrile to 38.9°C and tachycardic (heart rate, 116). She reported a tick bite 3 weeks prior. Peripheral blood smears, blood, and urine cultures were negative and her cerebrospinal fluid was normal. A CBC revealed a white blood cell (WBC) count of 7600 with 71% polymorphonuclear leukocytes and 16% neutrophils, a platelet count of 120,000 cells/μL, and elevated liver transaminases. The patient's chest radiograph was normal. However, she was admitted because of her septic appearance, and human anaplasmosis was presumptively diagnosed based on the clinical presentation and laboratory data. She was hydrated with intravenous (IV) fluids and started on IV doxycycline. A CBC the next day revealed WBC 6200 and platelets of 80,000 cells/μL. She improved within 24 hours and although her headaches persisted, she was discharged on oral doxycycline.

Blood taken before treatment was positive by PCR for *B miyamotoi* and negative for *A phagocytophilum* and *B microti*. At her outpatient follow-up, the patient stated that although her fever resolved within 24 hours of the IV doxycycline, she continued to have fatigue and headaches, unrelieved by oxycodone with acetaminophen. She was alert and oriented but complained of severe headache. Vital signs and physical examination were normal. She was advised to continue doxycycline for a period of 3 weeks and was given a prescription for butalbital/acetaminophen and caffeine for her headaches. She was re-evaluated 9 days later and all of her symptoms had resolved, including the headaches. A CBC drawn at that time showed a WBC 11,200/uL, hematocrit 42.8%, and platelets 397,000/μL. She has since remained well and is back to her normal activities.

Case 3. Recurrent Fever Presentation

A 57-year-old female nurse from southeastern Massachusetts felt ill at the end of July with generalized malaise and body aches. She is an avid gardener and has dogs, but did not recall any tick bites. None of her family members had been ill. Her past medical history is significant for hypertension and anxiety. She developed fevers, shaking chills, night sweats, and headaches and was evaluated in a local community hospital emergency room where she was given 2 L of IV fluids and sent home. She continued to be febrile with nausea, fatigue, and body aches and went to her primary care physician a few days later. A CBC demonstrated leukopenia and elevated transaminases. She gave a history of allergy to amoxicillin and tetracycline and was sent home without treatment. A whole-blood specimen was negative by PCR for *B microti* and *A phagocytophilum*, but serum was reactive for IgM-class antibodies to *B burgdorferi* using a whole-cell sonicate EIA, although confirmatory testing by immunoblot was negative. She continued to feel poorly with recurrent fever, chills, and headaches associated with anorexia and weight loss. She had multiple visits to her primary care provider, who continued to monitor her clinically with serial CBCs. No specific diagnosis was made.

Because of persistent symptoms, including fever, generalized arthralgias, malaise, headaches, nausea, and loss of appetite, the patient was examined by an infectious disease specialist approximately 5 to 6 weeks after her initial presentation. She stated her fevers resolved for several days and then relapsed, causing a recurrence of her symptom complex. Physical examination revealed an alert but pale and ill-looking woman. All other systems were unaffected and the patient was started on doxycycline while awaiting the results of the laboratory tests.

Blood samples drawn on August 2nd and August 30th yielded evidence of *B miyamotoi* DNA. She was re-evaluated on September 27th; the fever, headache, and joint pain had all resolved. She complained of extreme fatigue and the inability to function at her normal pace. Her examination at that visit was normal and her CBC had returned to normal values. She was advised to complete the 4 weeks of doxycycline given that she was able to tolerate it with no side effects. The patient called the office on October 16th stating all of her symptoms had resolved and she was feeling markedly better.

DIAGNOSIS

If Lyme disease is known to be zoonotic where the patient may have acquired infection, BMD is also likely to be endemic and thus should be considered in the differential diagnosis for a febrile, tick-exposed patient. As with the other deer tick–transmitted infections (ie, Lyme disease, babesiosis, human granulocytic ehrlichiosis [HGA], or Powassan/deer tick virus fever), patients with BMD present with an undifferentiated febrile illness, which may include acute headaches, fever, chills, myalgia, arthralgia, fatigue, or malaise. Patients with BMD often appear septic and laboratory studies reveal leukopenia, thrombocytopenia, and elevated transaminases. Such findings, along with clinical presentation, usually require providers to exclude HGA.

Specialized laboratory testing, particularly PCR testing of blood samples collected during acute infection and ideally before initiation of treatment, is useful for confirming a BMD diagnosis. Acute anticoagulated blood samples (EDTA or citrate, not heparin) taken before treatment may be analyzed for evidence of *B miyamotoi* DNA by PCR. Commercial testing laboratories are increasingly offering specific PCR testing for *B miyamotoi*, but physicians need to consider a clinical laboratory experience's with PCR in general when interpreting results. Like all other PCR assays, the failure to detect specific DNA or RNA in the blood does not exclude the possibility of BMD. In addition to *B burgdorferi*, concurrent infections with *B microti*, *A phagocytophilum*, or even deer tick virus are possible and should be ruled out.

Serology is a useful complementary method to PCR for confirming a BMD diagnosis.[12] Importantly, the recommended two-tiered serologic protocol[33] for confirming a *B burgdorferi* infection (EIA followed by immunoblot of reactive samples) is not useful for diagnosis of BMD. However, 23% of acute and 90% of convalescent sera from PCR-confirmed BMD cases were reactive for IgM antibodies to *B burgdorferi* using a sonicate antigen EIA. Few of these reactives were considered positive when immunoblots are interpreted as recommended.[34] No more than 20% of convalescent BMD sera were reactive in the IgG EIA and of these, only 7% were confirmed by immunoblot. Thus, an IgM reactive sample by Lyme enzyme-linked immunosorbent assay (ELISA), but not confirmed by immunoblot, may represent a response to *B miyamotoi* instead of *B burgdorferi*. Convalescent sera from patients with BMD rarely demonstrate IgG reactivity to *B burgdorferi* antigens.

The *B burgdorferi* EIA, when reactive for IgM but not confirmed for specific reactivity, may be effectively complemented by an EIA using a recombinant GlpQ protein. GlpQ is a 39- to 42-kDa protein that was identified by screening a *B hermsi* genomic library with high titered human sera collected from a patient with relapsing fever. GlpQ was demonstrated in all *Borrelia* spp examined except for *B burgdorferi* s.l., thus allowing for serologic discrimination of relapsing fever from Lyme disease.[35] More than 90% of convalescent sera from relapsing fever cases were reactive in EIAs using the rGlpQ protein, but none were reactive from either Lyme disease or syphilis cases. Given that *B miyamotoi* is more closely related to relapsing fever spirochetes than to *B burgdorferi* s.l., GlpQ was a natural target to serve as the basis for the development of an immunoassay to confirm a diagnosis of BMD.

The rGlpQ EIA seems to be sensitive and specific for confirming BMD.[12] Lyme disease patient sera did not react with rGlpQ, nor did those from patients with HGA or monocytic ehrlichiosis. A low frequency (14%) of IgM reactivity was observed with *B microti* patient sera; the biologic basis for this finding remains unexplored. Some (3.6%) serum samples from 250 healthy individuals residing west of the Mississippi River were considered IgG reactive; this puzzling finding may reflect exposure to relapsing fever spirochetes other than *B miyamotoi*. Although GlpQ homologs may be found in *Haemophilus influenzae* and even *Escherichia coli*, their sequences are divergent enough so that cross reactivity with *B miyamotoi* GlpQ is not likely.[13] Of a well-studied BMD case series, 86% were considered to have seroconverted to rGlpQ[12]; convalescent sera comprised those taken at least 5 days after initial presentation.

The need for a recombinant protein antigen was determined by the lack of availability of whole-cell *B miyamotoi* antigens. Although the Japanese *B miyamotoi* type strain HT31 was originally isolated in BSK II medium and apparently can be productively maintained *in vitro*, until very recently no one has succeeded in culturing the American or Eurasian strains. The only means of propagating these other strains has been by serial blood passage in SCID mice. These immunodeficient mice sustain spirochetemias approaching 1000 to 5000 bacteria/mL for long durations, and they are very useful in making primary isolates by inoculating blood from patients with BMD. However, the cost of purchasing SCID mice and maintaining them for the purpose of harvesting spirochetes for use as serologic reagents is prohibitive. HT31 itself is not available through American Type Culture Collection or other biologic repositories and must be requested from a handful of research laboratories within the United States or Europe.

Successful cultivation of *B miyamotoi* has recently been reported.[36,37] Both research groups report passaging HT31 and a North American *B miyamotoi* strain in variants of Kelly-Pettenkofer medium (Kelly medium is the base for BSK II medium, which is used to cultivate *B burgdorferi*). In one system, 10% fetal calf serum and slight modifications of the concentrations of bovine serum albumin, CMRL-1066 base, HEPES, glucose, and rabbit serum allowed for propagation within standard conditions used for *B burgdorferi*. In the other system, the critical factors included 50% fetal calf serum in a 6% carbon dioxide atmosphere. In both systems, cell densities did not exceed 10^7 bacteria/mL, whereas *B burgdorferi* in BSK II medium attains densities of 10^9 cells/mL.[32] Both research groups report failing to maintain *B miyamotoi* viability in unmodified BSKII medium but Fukunaga and colleagues[2] originally propagated HT31 in BSKII medium to densities sufficient to harvest cells for preparing immunoblots or DNA for Southern blots or pulse field gel electrophoresis. It may be that the three members of *B miyamotoi* s.l. may differ in their in vitro growth requirements, or that batches of BSK vary with respect to their capacity to sustain HT31 growth. In any event, the possibility of propagating *B miyamotoi* in vitro allows for generating more traditional serologic reagents, such as whole-cell sonicate EIAs and immunoblots.

SCID mice could be inoculated with acute blood samples and borreliae may be visualized by peripheral blood smears of the mice 7 to 14 days after inoculation (**Fig. 2**). The sensitivity of this procedure has not yet been determined and this method would be restricted to a limited number of research laboratories. Spirochetes were demonstrated in the cerebrospinal fluid of the American and European index cases, but these were unusual findings in elderly immunocompromised individuals. However, because *B miyamotoi* causes peripheral blood spirochetemia, Giemsa-stained blood smears made from acute blood samples may allow for a microscopic confirmation of the diagnosis. Thick smears, as performed for malaria diagnosis, are the most likely method for successful detection; by quantitative PCR, a range of 5 to 53,000 (mean, 8313) spirochetes were estimated per milliliter of whole blood from our recent case series.[12] For

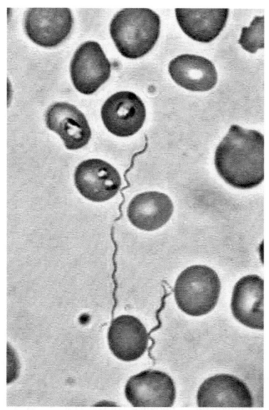

Fig. 2. Giemsa-stained (pH 7.0) thin blood smear of blood from a CB17-SCID mouse concurrently infected by *Babesia microti* and *Borrelia miyamotoi*. Three spirochetes are seen in this field (original magnification × 630), bright field illumination.

comparison, the sensitivity of thick blood smears for malarial parasites is approximately 15,000 infected red blood cells per milliliter.[38–40]

In summary, BMD should be considered in febrile patients from Lyme-endemic regions of the northeast United States, who present between April to November with evidence of a systemic illness or who appear septic. Other infections to be considered in these patients include Lyme disease without rash, babesiosis, HGA, deer tick virus fever, and West Nile fever. Elevated transaminases, leukopenia, and thrombocytopenia narrow the list of deer tick–transmitted infections to BMD and HGA; in sites with dog ticks or Lone Star ticks, rickettsiosis, monocytic ehrlichiosis, and tularemia may also be considered. PCR testing of an acute, pretreatment blood sample for *Borrelia* spp ("pan-borrelia"), preferably followed by a species specific PCR assay as a confirmatory identification, is the most efficient way to demonstrate active infection. As with Lyme disease or virtually any other tick-transmitted infection, acute serology for BMD is not sensitive, but it is useful as an archived comparison with a convalescent sample collected 3 to 4 weeks later. BMD convalescent serum is usually IgM reactive in *B burgdorferi* EIA (whole-cell sonicate), but the confirmatory Lyme immunoblot using the two-tiered protocol is not interpreted as positive. Only a fifth of convalescent BMD patient sera reacts in the *B burgdorferi* IgG EIA (and usually are negative by the confirmatory immunoblot), but more than 80% react in the rGlpQ EIA for IgG.

Hence, the confirmation of BMD rests on elevated transaminases, acute blood PCR, and seroconversion to rGlpQ.

TREATMENT

It is likely that BMD has been occurring in Lyme-endemic sites from the very beginning of our recognition of Lyme disease as an American zoonosis, but presumptively has been diagnosed as atypical Lyme disease and treated successfully on that basis. Oral doxycycline (100 mg twice a day for 10–21 days) or amoxicillin (500 mg three times a day for 14–21 days) as currently recommended for early disseminated Lyme disease[33] has been sufficient to treat BMD.[12] Treatment failure has not been documented. The clinical implications of milder infections and failure to treat remains undetermined; mild or subclinical infections clearly occur given the evidence for 5% to 10% prior exposure in New England communities suggested by cross-sectional serosurveys.[13] The manner in which BMD presents in children remains to be described.

Prevention is as for any other tick-borne infection, namely personal protection using repellents, such as DEET; clothing treatment with permethrin; daily showers; tick checks; prompt tick removal; and vigilance for unexplained fevers when living in or visiting Lyme-endemic sites.

SELF-ASSESSMENT

1. A patient presents during July with a 4-day history of fever, headache, myalgias, arthralgias, and fatigue. Laboratory studies are normal. The patient lives in a Lyme disease–endemic site and states that he frequently finds ticks on his dog. No rash is evident. Lyme disease is suspected and an ELISA screen for antibody to B burgdorferi is ordered. The ELISA is positive for IgM but not IgG; the IgM immunoblot confirmation test is negative, with only two of the three required bands observed. The health care provider can conclude which of the following:
   a. The patient likely has Lyme disease but the antibody response has not fully developed.
   b. The patient does not have Lyme disease because the immunoblot was negative.
   c. The patient may have either Lyme disease, or BMD, or both.
   d. Convalescent serology is indicated; the patient is treated presumptively for Lyme disease.
2. The physician diagnoses the previously described patient as having early Lyme disease and treats accordingly. The patient returns because he continues to experience fatigue and headache even after completing the first week of amoxicillin. The most appropriate follow-up is:
   a. PCR testing for B miyamotoi.
   b. Changing treatment to doxycycline.
   c. PCR testing for A phagocytophilum and B microti.
   d. Consider the IgM ELISA a false positive, stop the antibiotics, and suggest supportive care for undifferentiated viral illness.
3. You have been asked to speak in a public forum on preventing Lyme disease. You state that personal protection, such as repellents and tick checks, should be used from Memorial Day to Labor Day. The state public health epidemiologist demurs, saying that the months of greatest risk are June and July, and that repellent use is not without possible side effects. You justify your answer by:
   a. Noting that we need to take a holistic approach to preventing vector-borne infections and that mosquito transmitted infections are most common in August

and September. Deer ticks and dog ticks are most common in June and July. Thus, repellent use should be encouraged throughout the summer.
b. Agreeing that the months of greatest risk for Lyme disease are indeed June and July, but that some nymphal deer ticks are present in late May and even as late as August in most sites; and, that BMD may be transmitted by larvae, which are most common from July through September.
c. Stating that people are most active outdoors in Lyme endemic sites from Memorial Day to Labor Day and that any outdoor activity in sites where ticks are common should prompt personal protective efforts.
d. Disagreeing with the statement that repellent use is not without side effects; billions of doses of DEET have been applied with fewer than a few dozen known adverse events. The benefit of using repellent as directed by the product label far outweighs the small likelihood of harm caused by the repellent itself.

4. You see a patient with a 2-year history of nonspecific signs and symptoms, mainly fatigue and arthralgia. She has lived until recently in Manhattan, and admits to little outdoor activity. She has been diagnosed elsewhere with chronic Lyme disease and *Bartonella* coinfection, based on serologic testing at a specialty laboratory in California, and has been taking oral antibiotics for 7 months with no improvement. She requests PCR testing for BMD because she believes it could be yet another coinfection that is causing her illness. Your most appropriate action is:
a. Agree to evaluate her for BMD, because relatively little is known about this newly recognized infection.
b. Decline to order either PCR or serology for BMD, noting that all current information suggests that BMD is adequately treated using the typical regimens for Lyme disease and that there is no evidence for chronic sequelae.
c. Inform her that her illness cannot be BMD because some authorities suggest that *B miyamotoi* causes relapsing fever, and she does not report this.
d. Suggest that she have a general health work-up because her diagnosis of chronic Lyme disease with coinfection may be erroneous and is preventing the identification of other treatable conditions.

5. A patient who recently vacationed in northwest Wisconsin acutely presents with severe headache, fever, chills, and myalgia. The headache does not abate with over-the-counter analgesics. His CBC demonstrates leucopenia with left shift. Transaminases are slightly elevated. You suspect ehrlichiosis and presumptively treat with doxycycline. The headache and fever disappear 12 hours after the first 100-mg dose of doxycycline. The patient returns for a follow-up visit in 10 days, and a blood sample is drawn. The transaminases remain slightly elevated but the patient reports a full recovery. Serologies for specific antibody to *A phagocytophilum* and *Ehrlichia muris* are negative. You should consider:
a. The possibility that the ehrlichiosis diagnosis was incorrect, and order rGlpQ serology for BMD, and Lyme disease serology.
b. Nothing further. The patient was treated and reports full recovery. Confirming the diagnosis would only be useful for epidemiologic surveillance.
c. PCR and serologic testing for subclinical *B microti* infection because the patient is an avid blood donor and was very likely exposed to deer ticks; doxycycline would not have eliminated this protozoan and thus he might be a risk to the blood supply.
d. Nothing further: serology for confirming *A phagocytophilum* infection can be insensitive and prompt treatment may have blunted the antibody response.

Answers
Answer 1: A, C, and D are acceptable.
Answer 2: C
Answer 3: All are correct.
Answer 4: Either B or D.
Answer 5: Best answers are B or D; however, C might also be considered.

REFERENCES

1. Theiler A. Spirillosis of cattle. J Comp Pathol 1904;17:47–55.
2. Fukunaga M, Takahashi Y, Tsuruta Y, et al. Genetic and phenotypic analysis of *Borrelia miyamotoi* sp. nov., isolated from the ixodid tick *Ixodes persulcatus*, the vector for Lyme disease in Japan. Int J Syst Bacteriol 1995;45:804–10.
3. Armstrong PM, Rich SM, Smith RD, et al. A new borrelia infecting lone star ticks. Lancet 1996;347:67–8.
4. Barbour AG, Maupin GO, Teltow GJ, et al. Identification of an uncultivable *Borrelia* species in the hard tick, amblyomma americanum. J Infect Dis 1996;173:403–9.
5. Barbour AG. Phylogeny of a relapsing fever *Borrelia* species transmitted by the hard tick *Ixodes scapularis*. Infect Genet Evol 2014;27:551–8.
6. Callow LL. Observations on tick-transmitted spirochaetes of cattle in Australia and South Africa. Br Vet J 1967;123:492–7.
7. Smith RD, Miranpuri GS, Adams JH, et al. *Borrelia theileri*: isolation from ticks (*Boophilus microplus*) and tick-borne transmission between splenectomized calves. Am J Vet Res 1985;46:1396–8.
8. Feder HM Jr, Hoss DM, Zemel L, et al. Southern tick-associated rash illness (STARI) in the north: STARI following a tick bite in Long Island, New York. Clin Infect Dis 2011;53:e142–6.
9. Platonov AE, Karan LS, Kolyasnikova NM, et al. Humans infected with relapsing fever spirochete *Borrelia miyamotoi*, Russia. Emerg Infect Dis 2011;17:1816–23.
10. Gugliotta JL, Goethert HK, Berardi VP, et al. Meningoencephalitis from *Borrelia miyamotoi* in an immunocompromised patient. N Engl J Med 2013;368:240–5.
11. Hovius JWR, de Wever B, Sohne M, et al. A case of meningoencephalitis by the relapsing fever spirochete *Borrelia miyamotoi* in Europe. Lancet 2013;382:658.
12. Molloy PJ, Telford SR, Chowdri HR, et al. *Borrelia miyamotoi* disease in the northeastern United States: a case series. Ann Intern Med 2015;163(2):91–8.
13. Krause PJ, Narasimhan S, Wormser GP, et al. *Borrelia miyamotoi* sensu lato seroreactivity and seroprevalence in the northeastern United States. Emerg Infect Dis 2014;20:1183–90.
14. Fillipova NA. Taiga tick: *Ixodes persulcatus schulze* (acarina: ixodidae). Leningrad (Russia): Nauka Publishers; 1985. p. 416.
15. Bacon RM, Kugeler KJ, Mead PS. Surveillance for Lyme disease—United States, 1992-2006. MMWR Surveill Summ 2008;57(SS10):1–9.
16. Scoles GA, Papero MA, Beati L, et al. A relapsing fever group spirochete transmitted by *Ixodes scapularis* ticks. Vector Borne Zoonotic Dis 2001;1:21–34.
17. Richter D, Schlee DB, Matuschka FR. Relapsing fever-like spirochetes infecting European vector tick of Lyme disease agent. Emerg Infect Dis 2003;9:697–701.
18. Mun J, Eisen RJ, Eisen L, et al. Detection of a *Borrelia miyamotoi* sensu lato relapsing-fever group spirochete from *Ixodes pacificus* in California. J Med Entomol 2006;43:120–3.

19. Ogden NH, Margos G, Aanensen DM, et al. Investigation of genotypes of *Borrelia burgdorferi* in *Ixodes scapularis* ticks collected during surveillance in Canada. Appl Environ Microbiol 2011;77:3244–54.
20. Barbour AG, Bunikis J, Travinsky B, et al. Niche partitioning of *Borrelia burgdorferi* and *Borrelia miyamotoi* in the same tick vector and mammalian reservoir species. Am J Trop Med Hyg 2009;81:1120–31.
21. Burri C, Schumann O, Schumann C, et al. Are *Apodemus* spp. mice and *Myodes glareolus* reservoirs for *Borrelia miyamotoi, Candidatus Neoehrlichia mikurensis, Rickettsia helvetica, R. monacensis* and *Anaplasma phagocytophilum*? Ticks Tick Borne Dis 2014;5:245–51.
22. Taylor KR, Takano A, Konnai S, et al. *Borrelia miyamotoi* infections among wild rodents show age and month independence and correlation with *Ixodes persulcatus* larval attachment in Hokkaido, Japan. Vector Borne Zoonotic Dis 2013;13:92–7.
23. Hamer SA, Hickling GJ, Keith R, et al. Associations of passerine birds, rabbits, and ticks with *Borrelia miyamotoi* and *Borrelia andersonii* in Michigan, U.S.A. Parasit Vectors 2012;5:231.
24. Rollend L, Fish D, Childs JE. Transovarial transmission of *Borrelia* spirochetes by *Ixodes scapularis*: a summary of the literature and recent observations. Ticks Tick Borne Dis 2013;4:46–51.
25. Burgdorfer W, Varma MGR. Transstadial and transovarial development of disease agents in arthropods. Annu Rev Entomol 1967;12:347–76.
26. Spencer RR, Parker RR. Rocky mountain spotted fever: infectivity of fasting and recently fed ticks. Publ Health Rep 1923;38:333.
27. Katavolos P, Armstrong PM, Dawson JE, et al. Duration of tick attachment required for transmission of human granulocytic ehrlichiosis. J Infect Dis 1998;177:1422–5.
28. Rosa PA, Tilly K, Stewart PE. The burgeoning molecular genetics of the Lyme disease spirochaete. Nat Rev Microbiol 2005;3:129–43.
29. Krause PJ, Hendrickson JE, Steeves TK, et al. Blood transfusion transmission of the tick-borne relapsing fever spirochete *Borrelia miyamotoi* in mice. Transfusion 2015;55:593–7.
30. Chowdri HR, Gugliotta JL, Berardi VP, et al. *Borrelia miyamotoi* infection presenting as human granulocytic anaplasmosis: a case report. Ann Intern Med 2013;159:21–7.
31. Southern P, Sanford J. Relapsing fever. A clinical and microbiological review. Medicine 1969;48:129–49.
32. Barbour AG. Immunobiology of relapsing fever. Contrib Microbiol Immunol 1987;8:125–7.
33. Wormser GP, Dattwyler RJ, Shapiro ED, et al. The clinical assessment, treatment, and prevention of Lyme disease, human granulocytic anaplasmosis, and babesiosis: clinical practice guidelines by the infectious diseases society of America. Clin Infect Dis 2006;43:1089–134.
34. Centers for Disease Control and Prevention. Recommendations for test performance from the second national conference on serologic diagnosis of Lyme disease. MMWR Surveill Summ 1995;44:590–1.
35. Schwan TG, Schrumpf ME, Hinnebusch BJ, et al. GlpQ: an antigen for serological discrimination between relapsing fever and Lyme borreliosis. J Clin Microbiol 1996;34:2483–92.
36. Wagemakers A, Oei A, Fikrig MM, et al. The relapsing fever spirochete *Borrelia miyamotoi* is cultivable in a modified Kelly-Pettenkofer medium, and is resistant to human complement. Parasit Vectors 2014;7:418.

37. Margos G, Stockmeier S, Hizo-Teufel C, et al. Long-term in vitro cultivation of *Borrelia miyamotoi*. Ticks Tick Borne Dis 2015;6:181–4.
38. Bruce Chwatt LJ. Essential malariology. 2nd edition. New York: John Wiley and Sons; 1985. p. 452.
39. Pollack RJ, Telford SR III, Spielman A. Standardisation of a complex medium for the growth of *Borrelia burgdorferi*. J Clin Microbiol 1993;31:1251–5.
40. Telford SR, Goethert HK. Emerging and emergent tick borne infections. In: Chappell LH, Bowman AS, Nuttall PA, editors. Ticks: biology, disease and control. Cambridge, UK: Cambridge University Press; 2008. p. 344–76.

Methods to Prevent Tick Bites and Lyme Disease

Nick H. Ogden, DPhil[a],*, L. Robbin Lindsay, PhD[b], Steven W. Schofield, PhD[c]

KEYWORDS

- Personal protection • Lyme disease • Repellent • *Ixodes scapularis*
- *Ixodes pacificus*

KEY POINTS

- There are no licensed vaccines for protection of humans against Lyme disease. Prevention thus relies on the following:
  - Avoiding areas where ticks that transmit *Borrelia burgdorferi* occur, at times that the ticks are active.
  - Personal prevention of tick bites and transmission of *B burgdorferi* through wearing of appropriate clothing, use of insect repellents and clothing treatments, and prompt removal of unattached or attached ticks before they respectively attach to feed or transmit *B burgdorferi* while feeding.
  - Reducing environmental risk by controlling ticks and tick infections with pesticide applications; reservoir-targeted interventions (eg, bait boxes); and landscape management.
  - Prophylactic treatment with antibiotics after a tick bite to prevent transmitted *B burgdorferi* from producing clinical Lyme disease.

INTRODUCTION

Lyme disease occurs in 3 main regions of North America: (i) the US Pacific coast states and southern British Columbia in Canada, where the main vector is the western blacklegged tick, *Ixodes pacificus*; (ii) the contiguous US upper Midwest/southern Manitoba/Northwestern Ontario; and (iii) the contiguous US mid-Atlantic and northeastern states/southeastern Canada. In the latter 2 regions, the blacklegged tick, *Ixodes scapularis*, is the vector.[1,2] It is this species that is associated with the large

Disclosure Statement: The authors have nothing to disclose.
Conflict of Interest: The authors have no conflicts of interests to declare.
[a] National Microbiology Laboratory, Public Health Agency of Canada, 3200 Sicotte, Saint-Hyacinthe, Quebec J2S 7C6, Canada; [b] National Microbiology Laboratory, Public Health Agency of Canada, 1015 Arlington Street, Winnipeg, Manitoba R3E 3R2, Canada; [c] Communicable Disease Control Program, Force Health Protection, Department of National Defence, 1745 Alta Vista Drive, Ottawa, Ontario K1A 0K6, Canada
* Corresponding author.
E-mail address: nicholas.ogden@phac-aspc.gc.ca

Clin Lab Med 35 (2015) 883–899
http://dx.doi.org/10.1016/j.cll.2015.07.003
labmed.theclinics.com

majority of Lyme disease cases as well the increase in the numbers of cases reported over recent decades.[3,4] The key role of this species reflects its recent significant geographic range expansion (northward, westward, and southward) out from refuges in the northeastern and upper Midwestern United States, so many more people now live in areas where this species occurs.[3,4] Also, this vector usually has higher infection prevalence than does *I pacificus*. Accordingly, the risk associated with a bite from this vector is usually higher. This is not to say that infection prevalence is always high for this species: *I scapularis* occurs widely in the southern and southeastern United States, where it is rarely infected with *Borrelia burgdorferi*.[5]

Given the increasing threat of Lyme disease, the need for effective methods to protect against this disease has never been greater.[6,7] Options in this regard are limited, not least because there are no licensed human vaccines against Lyme disease and area-wide and centrally organized tick control programs are lacking.[8] Nevertheless, exposure to ticks and *B burgdorferi* can be reduced, usually at the individual person or individual property level, with several relatively simple interventions[9-13]:

- Avoiding areas where ticks that transmit *B burgdorferi* occur, at times that the ticks are active;
- Applying personal protective measures, such as wearing appropriate clothing, using insect repellents and clothing treatments, and removing ticks before they can attach and transmit *B burgdorferi*;
- Reducing environmental risk by controlling ticks and tick infections with pesticide applications; reservoir-targeted interventions (eg, bait boxes); and landscape management;
- Using prophylactic antibiotics in an appropriate manner after a tick bite to prevent transmitted *B burgdorferi* from producing clinical Lyme disease.

The target audience for this review includes medical professionals who provide advice on Lyme disease and its prevention, and public health professionals who may wish to use and disseminate this information.

Avoiding Risk Areas

A simple rule for Lyme disease is: "if you don't get a tick, you don't get sick." In recent times in the United States, and currently in many parts of Canada, this could be achieved by avoiding the areas where Lyme disease occurs.[1,14,15] The range expansion of *I scapularis* and Lyme disease has changed this, and these ticks are now found in more regions and have also moved into more densely populated areas, including on or close to private/residential properties.[16] Nonetheless, avoidance can be a viable risk-reduction approach—at least in some locations and situations.[12]

So how can ticks and Lyme disease be avoided? First, ticks are associated with specific habitats, in particular, mixed wooded areas that support the rodent, bird, and deer hosts of the ticks.[17-19] In these habitats, ticks often are found in leaf litter, at the edges (ecotone) of forested habitats, as well as along hiking or animal trails.[19] Tick populations can exist in quite small patches of woodland, including those found in backyards, but are less frequently encountered on lawns, especially those that are kept short.[20-22] Thus, if woodland leaf litter and ecotone habitats can be avoided, the risk of tick bites is generally very low.[23] Conversely, visiting such habitats increases exposure and should prompt consideration of use of additional interventions.

Second, the risk of bites and Lyme disease is higher in areas where ticks are established (ie, are self-sustaining).[24,25] This is not to say that exposure cannot occur in other areas. Small numbers of adventitious ticks can occur outside areas where tick populations have become established due to dispersal by mammal and bird hosts.[14,26] However, avoiding areas where tick populations are established will reduce (but may not totally eliminate) risk. Federal, state, and provincial public health Web sites frequently provide information on where the ticks have become established.

Third, risk varies by season. It is highest in the spring and summer months (May through August) when nymphal ticks are active.[27,28] This life stage presents a higher risk than adult ticks for at least 2 reasons: nymphs are more abundant (so the likelihood of being bitten by a tick is much higher), and they are smaller and harder to find, which heightens the probability that they will feed long enough to transmit B burgdorferi. This timing is critical, because the duration of tick feeding is an important factor in B burgdorferi transmission. There is a latent period of 48 to 72 hours between the tick starting to feed and it being capable of transmitting B burgdorferi due to B burgdorferi residing in the gut of the unfed infected tick. Once the tick starts to feed, B burgdorferi begins to multiply, penetrates the tick's gut wall, and then migrates to the salivary glands from where it is delivered into the host. This process usually takes 48 to 72 hours and if attached ticks are removed before 48 hours transmission will be prevented in most cases.[29] Risk does exist earlier in the spring and into the autumn when adult ticks are active.[17] Although larval ticks will occasionally bite people, they are not infected with B burgdorferi and hence do not present a risk of Lyme disease. Avoiding risk areas during the times of year that nymphs and adult ticks are active will significantly reduce or eliminate exposure.[30] However, it should be noted that adult ticks can sometimes be active and potentially transmit Lyme disease through cooler periods, for example, when temperatures are above freezing and snow is not on the ground.[19,31]

Preventing Bites and Pathogen Transmission

If avoidance of tick habitats is not possible, then risk reduction relies on preventing bites or by promptly removing attached ticks before they have time to transmit B burgdorferi. These personal protective approaches are summarized in **Table 1**.

Table 1
Methods for preventing tick bites or pathogen transmission

Strategy/Method	Rationale for Use	Selected References
Avoid tick-infested habitats	Prevents exposure to ticks	12,25
Wear appropriate clothing, eg, light-colored and long-sleeve shirts, socks, and full trousers	Limits or delays access by ticks to sites for attachment and improves ability to detect (and remove) unattached ticks on clothing	40
Use approved, topical repellents (DEET or picaridin) on skin; wear insecticide-treated clothing (where permitted)	Prevents ticks from biting; some products can kill ticks	33,113,114
Do tick checks at least once a day; remove any ticks that are found	Removes tick before transmission of the pathogen can occur	54,115
Bath or shower soon after leaving tick habitat, eg, within 2 h	May dislodge unattached ticks; provides additional opportunity to find/remove attached ticks	49

Data from Refs.[12,25,33,40,49,54,113–115]

Use of topical repellents

Repellents prevent the bites of many arthropod vectors, including ticks.[32,33] They function through their direct effect on the sensory apparatus of the host-seeking arthropod.[33] Both the US Centers for Disease Control and Prevention (CDC) and the Public Health Agency of Canada (PHAC) recommend the use of repellents to prevent tick bites.[4,34] Moreover, these agencies are similar in that they specifically recommend the active ingredient N,N-diethyl-meta-toluamide (DEET) for this purpose.[2,34,35] PHAC also recommends picaridin (called icaridin in Canada) for the prevention of tick bites; both agencies tend to favor products that contain 20% to 30% DEET or 20% picaridin because they provide longer periods of protection against ticks and other arthropod bites.[36] In Canada, children less than 12 years of age are only permitted to use products that contain 10% or less DEET, whereas there are no age-based limits for picaridin.[35,36] Other repellent options for prevention of bites include IR3535 and oil of lemon eucalyptus/p-methane-3, 8-diol in the United States and Canada.[37–39] Importantly, all products registered in the United States (by the Environmental Protection Agency [EPA]) and Canada (by Health Canada) have been subjected to a stringent regulatory evaluation, and hence, have a favorable safety profile. The corollary is that products that have not been subjected to this process, including those purported to be natural, might present unacceptable risks—whether because they fail to prevent bites or because they have not been adequately screened for safety.

Wear appropriate clothing

Blacklegged ticks typically wait on emergent vegetation (eg, grasses or shrubs) or leaf litter, and then grab onto a host when it moves near.[19] If appropriate clothing is worn, which includes long trousers, socks, and long shirts, it should limit points of access for ticks to the underlying skin.[40] Furthermore, if ticks are forced to travel longer distances on outer garments, they might be more easily spotted and removed before attachment. Light-colored clothing might help in this regard.[41] If there is concern that clothing is contaminated with ticks, washing and drying (on high heat) can be used to sterilize the garments of ticks.[42]

Clothing treatments

Clothing treated with permethrin protects against tick bites.[43–46] Permethrin has direct effects on the nervous system of arthropods and hence can kill then directly, cause "knock-down," or elicit behavioral changes that result in the arthropod leaving the host. For ticks, permethrin-treated attire is sometimes characterized as being particularly efficacious.[33] This finding is supported by a recent randomized controlled trial that demonstrated treated clothing had greater than 80% protective efficacy against Amblyomma americanum ticks during the first year of use among occupationally exposed outdoors workers.[47] In the United States, permethrin-treated clothing and clothing treatments are commercially available for use by the public, including children. Moreover, it is specifically recommended for protection against tick bites, in the United States and abroad.[34,48] In Canada, permethrin on clothing is recommended for Canadians traveling abroad, including to Lyme disease-endemic areas in the United States.[33] However, clothing treatments are not licensed for use in Canada (except by the military) and hence are not widely available. The exceptions are travel health specialists who are permitted to sell treated products (or treatments) to Canadians traveling internationally.

Importantly, *only* products approved for the specific purpose of treating clothing to prevent tick and mosquito bites should be used. Use of other products that contain permethrin (or other insecticides) might result in untoward effects, whether due to substandard efficacy or excess chemical exposure.

Tick checks

Blacklegged ticks feed on their human hosts for up to 7 days.[19] As mentioned above, transmission of *B burgdorferi* does not occur immediately; rather, it takes a day or more to happen. Therefore, removal of ticks within a day or so will usually prevent transmission. This prevention of transmission is supported by epidemiologic studies, where carrying out a daily tick check (ie, explicitly checking one's body for ticks) or bathing or showering within 2 hours of outdoor activity (which increases the chances of finding ticks) reduced the risk of Lyme disease.[49] Rates of Lyme disease in placebo groups in studies evaluating the efficacy of prophylaxis after tick bite also provide indirect support for this approach: the risk of study participants that had a tick bite developing Lyme disease even if they received a placebo was very low (<1%) if the tick was removed rapidly, but if the tick that fed on them showed signs of engorgement (ie, had fed for several days), the probability of a person acquiring Lyme disease was markedly higher (~10%).[50] Usually, a tick check would be done after leaving a risk area, although it also is prudent to check for ticks that might be moving over clothing or skin while in tick habitats, although this would seem to be rarely done by exposed persons.[51]

Removal of attached ticks is ideally done with fine-tipped, stiff, and angled forceps (tweezers) placed around the head of the tick as near as is possible to the skin, followed by a steady, upward pulling movement[52–55] (**Fig. 1**). After the tick is removed, the bite site should be cleaned with soap and water and treated with an antiseptic.

Effectiveness of personal protection

The personal protection methods described in this section rely on individuals to use them. Although evidence supports their efficacy in preventing tick bites, it is often not clear that they are effective for the prevention of Lyme disease. To an extent, this reflects a relative absence of evidence demonstrating direct impact on Lyme disease incidence. However, the authors suggest that protection against bites, while indirect, is a reasonable proxy for protection against Lyme disease. More problematic is the issue of adherence, which often is low, whether for protection against ticks or more generally against hematophagous arthropods.[56–59] A recently published study from a nationwide, cross-sectional survey that was designed to be nationally representative based on US Census Bureau demographics reported that 51.2% of respondents did not take any routine personal prevention measures against tick exposure during warm

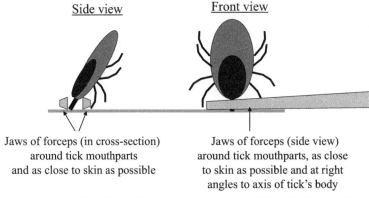

Side view   Front view

Jaws of forceps (in cross-section)   Jaws of forceps (side view)
around tick mouthparts   around tick mouthparts, as close
and as close to skin as possible   to skin as possible and at right
angles to axis of tick's body

Fig. 1. A recommended method of grasping an attached tick with forceps that permits removal with the least chance of crushing the tick or leaving the tick mouthparts in the skin.

weather.[60] There are a myriad of explanations for poor adherence, ranging from inconvenience, to concern about product safety, to perceptions and beliefs about the threat of Lyme disease. Unfortunately, there are no clear solutions to this problem. Education and encouragement are prudent, but it remains unclear if such efforts will meaningfully impact adherence and prevention of Lyme disease.[58]

Reducing Environmental Risk

Strategies for reducing risk of exposure to infected ticks in the environment are typically designed to reduce the abundance of ticks and the proportion of ticks that are infected with *B burgdorferi*. Currently, these include application of pesticides, including biological pesticides, to tick habitats or onto host animals, reduction of host animal populations, and modifications of the local landscapes in order to reduce their suitability for ticks and their natural hosts. Most of these measures are used in the peridomestic setting, and most are initiated by, and benefit, individual home or property owners, although they also can provide community level control.[9]

Use of pesticides to control ticks

In the United States, there are several different active ingredients registered for the control of ticks; however, those containing synthetic pyrethroids (which act in a way similar to permethrin) are most commonly used.[61] Application typically is onto vegetation and is done by homeowners or commercial applicators in areas where ticks occur, primarily in transition areas between woodlands and lawns. These treatments can substantially reduce tick populations.[9,62,63] In one study, a single well-timed treatment achieved a 90% reduction.[61] However, use of pesticides for tick control is not widespread, perhaps because of concern about safety or cost.[57] The development or refinement of novel products with less potential for nontarget impacts (eg, insecticidal soaps, desiccants, natural plant extracts like nootkatone) might enhance use, although cost and the potential need for repeat treatments will remain constraints.[64–67]

Another approach to controlling ticks with pesticides is direct treatment of white-tailed deer (the main host species for adult ticks) and rodents (the main reservoir of *B burgdorferi*) at bait stations. These techniques have shown efficacy in some studies, but not in others. For example, deployment of the 4-poster deer feeding station in northeastern United States significantly reduced nymphal blacklegged tick populations in 6 of 7 states, and by the sixth treatment year, the relative density of nymphal populations were reduced by 71% (range: 60%–82%).[68] Similarly, in a 3-year study in Connecticut, use of modified commercial bait boxes treated with Fipronil resulted in a 53% reduction in *B burgdorferi* infection prevalence in white-footed mice, 50% and 77% reductions in the abundance of host-seeking nymphs and adults, respectively, as well as a 67% reduction in *B burgdorferi* infection prevalence in nymphal ticks.[69] In contrast, a 5-year study of the 4-poster devices in Massachusetts reduced host-seeking tick populations by less than 10% and use of permethrin-treated bedding to control ticks on rodents provided significant tick reductions in Massachusetts but not at sites in Connecticut and New York.[70,71] Although promising, use of pesticides in these ways remains largely experimental, without wide adoption outside the research setting. Moreover, in some jurisdictions, treatment of deer might not be permitted or desirable because bait stations could act as a nexus for enhanced transmission of other infectious diseases like chronic wasting disease.[72]

Management of tick hosts including reservoirs

A significant amount of work has been done on control of ticks through host removal and exclusion techniques. In general, the diversity of hosts used by immature blacklegged ticks significantly hampers this approach for these life stages.[73] In contrast, management of white-tailed deer, which are a critical host for adult ticks, has been shown to impact tick populations.[74] However, the evidence suggests that deer populations must be markedly reduced (ie, fewer than 7 deer per square kilometer[75]) and that reductions must be sustained if a measurable impact on tick populations is to be achieved,[76,77] thus limiting the utility of deer control. Indeed, it might be best used as a niche technique in areas with a closed population of deer, for example, on islands.[78] A further limitation is opposition to deer removal, in particular, if achieved through a hunting-based cull.[79,80] Likely more palatable is exclusion through use of fencing, a technique that has been demonstrated to markedly reduce tick populations within large and small (<1 ha) fenced areas.[81–83] Although the perception of reduced environmental impact with fencing might be attractive when compared with other options, the cost of purchasing, installing, and maintaining fencing can be substantial.[61]

Dogs can acquire Lyme disease but are not known to act as reservoirs and cannot directly transmit infection to humans. Despite a small number of studies that suggest dog ownership does not increase an owner's risk of Lyme disease, pets (dogs and cats) could carry ticks acquired in woodlands into the home or yard.[84–86] It is thus prudent to routinely treat pets with tick control agents, whether applied externally or taken as an oral medication, if pets are regularly exposed to high-risk areas.[86,87] Only products that have been approved for use on pets should be used.

Recently, vaccination of wild rodent reservoirs against the outer surface protein A (OspA) of *B burgdorferi* has been suggested as a means to reduce the prevalence of infection in host-seeking ticks.[88] However, this approach has only shown modest impact in experimental studies where a single host was targeted.[89] It is likely that the complex ecology of Lyme disease limits impact when vaccination targets a single host.[90,91] However, it is possible that targeting a broader range of potential reservoir hosts might enhance impact.

Vegetation or landscape management

Vegetation or landscape management is a simple intervention that can reduce the suitability of areas to ticks or their hosts. Blacklegged ticks typically live within deciduous forests and require high humidity in their immediate microhabitat to survive.[17,92] Simple techniques like removal of brush and leaf litter reduce habitat suitability and have been shown to reduce tick populations.[93,94] Prescribed burning of vegetation can also reduce blacklegged tick populations, although reductions, if they occur, are usually short lived.[71,95,96] Furthermore, burning has limited application in more densely populated localities where Lyme disease is a threat.[71]

Other landscaping approaches can be used to decrease the suitability of residential properties for ticks. These approaches include removal of specific plants associated with increased tick abundance like Japanese Barberry; use of herbage that is less attractive to deer such as ferns, native grasses, and unpalatable tree species such as spruce; and desiccant barriers (gravel or wood chips) at the boundary of high- (forest edge) and low-risk zones (lawns).[71,97] Finally, tick unfriendly zones can be created by integrating landscape structures (eg, a raised deck) and management practices (eg, grass cutting, scrub removal, xeriscaping). An excellent summary of vegetation management for tick control is provided in Ref.[61]

Biological control

There are several biological control agents that can be used against blacklegged ticks, including nematodes, a wasp parasitoid (*Ixodiphagus hookeri*), and several species of fungi.[61] The fungi, *Metarhizium anisopliae* (strain F52) and *Beauveria bassiana*, have been evaluated against blacklegged ticks and *M anisopliae* has been registered by the EPA for use in the United States.[98] Unlike chemical pesticides, the efficacy of these fungicides to reduce tick abundance can vary widely among study sites and within and between years.[98,99] Tick abundance is usually reduced by 50% to 60% compared with untreated sites, but reductions greater than 85% have been reported. Applications of *M anisopliae* can effectively reduce tick numbers on residential lawns (56%) and in forested edge habitats (85%).[98] Some of the variability in control efficacy is likely due to environmental parameters, such as low relative humidity, high temperatures, precipitation, and solar ultraviolet radiation, which can have detrimental effects on spore viability, persistence, and efficacy.[98] Thus, although use of fungi-based biocontrol is promising, more work is needed to fully characterize its utility.[100] Finally, although birds like helmeted guineafowl are anecdotally reported as avid predators of blacklegged ticks and hence are put forward as good biocontrol agents, their impact has been very modest in controlled studies.[101]

Effectiveness of tick control

For most tick-control strategies, efficacy at reducing tick populations is readily demonstrable over a short time period (days or weeks). The larger challenge, however, is achieving longer-term reductions and ultimately achieving reductions in Lyme disease incidence. These outcomes remain elusive. This problem is underscored by the work of Hinckley and colleagues,[102] whereby a single treatment of a pesticide reduced tick abundance by 48% to 76%, but without an impact on reported tick attachments to human hosts or incidence of Lyme disease. Clearly, more work using direct patient important outcomes, for example tick attachment or clinical Lyme disease, are needed. Furthermore, a greater emphasis should be placed on use of multiple methods, ideally applied at a community scale, for tick control. As for mosquito control, community approaches are more likely to be effective than control applied at the level of the individual property.[9,12]

Human vaccines against Lyme disease

An effective vaccine would be a very valuable tool in the attempts to prevent Lyme disease. A vaccine marketed under the name LYMErix (SmithKlineBeecham, Pittsburgh, PA, USA) was available in the United States and Canada. It was developed in the early 1990s using recombinant OspA of *B burgdorferi*. The vaccine was approximately 80% effective at preventing new infections in adults.[103] It was approved by the FDA in 1998, but was withdrawn 3 years later because of (ill-founded) concerns that it stimulated autoantibody production.[103] Vaccine development research has recently been reinvigorated, with exploration of OspA, OspC (outer surface protein C), and combination subunits as antigens.[104] However, it is unlikely that a commercial product will be available in North America in the near future.

Prophylactic Treatment for Those Bitten by Ticks

Clinical Lyme disease can be prevented by taking antibiotic prophylaxis after receiving a tick bite.[50,105–108] There is, however, uncertainty in how to best use post-bite prophylaxis (PBP). Most people who receive a tick bite will not go on to develop disease, and, even in areas where tick infection rates are high, it is estimated that approximately 50 people must be treated to prevent a case of Lyme disease.[108] Furthermore, there are potential harms associated with treatment including direct effects on patients (eg, an estimated 1 case of nausea per 6.7 persons treated with doxycycline) and possible indirect impacts of widespread use on antimicrobial resistance.

The most widely accepted guideline on clinical management of Lyme disease, from the Infectious Diseases Society of America (IDSA), takes a conservative approach and recommends against routine use of PBP.[109] However, it allows that, if indicators suggestive of a high-risk bite are met (ie, exposure in an area where tick infection rates are $\geq$20%, bite from a vector tick, tick removed no more than 72 hours before treatment can begin, tick attached for 36 hours; **Table 2**), then prophylaxis with a single dose of doxycycline *may be offered* (if not contraindicated). The advantage of this algorithm is that it focuses prophylaxis on those at highest risk for developing clinical disease. A cost of this approach, however, is reduced sensitivity—some people who are excluded from treatment will go on to develop Lyme disease. The guidelines also do not explicitly consider patient values and preferences, an aspect that is becoming increasingly important to evidence-based medicine.[110] The consideration of patient values and preferences is relevant because the authors suspect that some (perhaps many) patients would place a relatively higher value on avoiding a small risk of Lyme disease (and associated worry) through use of a single dose of doxycycline than on the risk of the generally mild adverse events associated with PBP. Consider the case of a patient who removes an engorged tick acquired in a location where infection prevalence is 15% and then seeks (within 72 hours) medical attention. This situation meets most of the IDSA criteria, but not the prevalence threshold of 20%. Hence, if the guidelines were followed to the letter, this patient would not be offered PBP even though their risk of developing Lyme disease is for all intents and purposes similar to a patient receiving a similar bite and who is offered PBP because infection prevalence meets the 20% threshold. Perhaps more difficult are situations where some of the IDSA criteria are impossible (eg, a tick is not available, or infection prevalence is unknown) or difficult to assess (ie, duration of tick attachment), or where a patient strongly desires treatment for a risk assessed as relatively low.[111,112] For these patients, the IDSA guideline provides a powerful foundation for assessing the relative threat associated with a given exposure, which in turn can be used to inform decision-making related to PBP. For example, where there is no objective evidence that a bite has occurred, where a vector tick has been recovered but has likely been feeding for 24 hours or less, or where a tick

| Table 2 | |
| Criteria for assessing the risk of Lyme disease associated with a tick bite | |
Criteria	Factors Influencing Certainty of Criteria
Attached tick can be reliably identified as an adult female or nymphal blacklegged tick	Sometimes local knowledge is limited on tick species biting people
Female or nymphal tick has been attached for $\geq$36 h (based on level of engorgement or exposure history of patient)	Limited local knowledge of the relative size or appearance of feeding ticks, equipment to score the level of engorgement (dissecting microscope or hand lens) may not be available in some circumstances
Prophylaxis can be started within 72 h of the time that the tick was removed	No uncertainty presuming person can provide an accurate exposure history
Ecological information indicates that the local rates of infection with *B burgdorferi* in host-seeking ticks is $\geq$20%	Attending physician may not have access to these data or they have not been compiled for the region/city or town where the tick thesewas most likely to have been acquired

Adapted from Wormser GP, Dattwyler RJ, Shapiro ED, et al. The clinical assessment, treatment, and prevention of Lyme disease, human granulocytic anaplasmosis, and babesiosis: clinical practice guidelines by the Infectious Diseases Society of America. Clin Infect Dis 2006;43(9):1089–134.

bite has been acquired in the southeastern United States, both risk and the utility of PBP are likely negligible. In contrast, a bite from a known vector in a hyperendemic area, but with uncertainty about feeding status/duration, carries greater risk and hence also greater potential benefit to using PBP.

Clearly, risk assessment and decision-making for PBP are predicated on the knowledge and skills of the health care provider and open communication between the medical professional and the patient. For the provider, an ability to quickly identify (or to have identified) ticks is important, as is a capability to estimate duration of attachment based on physical observation (fed vs unfed) and a careful assessment of case history. Knowledge of tick ecology can also be useful, because tick attachments in the autumn are likely adult blacklegged ticks in some areas (because few other species are active at this time). In these same areas, and earlier in the season, including during the summer months when nymphs are prevalent, other tick species are also active and a tick bite (in the absence of a specimen) cannot be reliably ascribed to exposure to blacklegged ticks. The bottom line is that applying ecological information/knowledge can help to refine assessments of risk and ultimately should lead to a more informed discussion/decision related to use (or not) of PBP.

Recommendations

In areas where exposure cannot be otherwise avoided, the following preventive approaches are recommended:

- Use topical repellent (ie, that contains DEET or picaridin) on exposed areas of skin or clothing. Follow the instructions provided on the label of the repellent;
- Cover-up with appropriate clothing. If feasible, wash (and dry) clothing after spending time in risk areas;
- Where permitted, use insecticide-treated clothing;
- When in areas of risk, carry out tick checks at least on a daily basis. Where possible, shower or bathe within a few hours after leaving areas where ticks are thought to occur;
- Remove attached ticks with forceps (tweezers);
- Consider managing tick populations through landscape modification or use of pesticides, ideally at the community level.

SELF-ASSESSMENT

1. In which of the following areas is risk of Lyme disease minimal/absent?
   a. Minnesota
   b. Southern/Southeastern United States
   c. New England
   d. South Eastern Canada
2. Which of the following activities would not be considered a typical risk factor for exposure to blacklegged ticks?
   a. Cutting brush in a wooded area
   b. Jogging/running on a well-maintained and wide hard-packed trail
   c. Hunting
   d. Hiking
3. Which of the following is considered a useful method of personal protection?
   a. Removal of attached ticks by burning, or application of caustic substances
   b. Homeopathic nosodes
   c. Use of nonapproved (including natural) repellents
   d. Showering after outdoor activities

4. In which of the following scenarios is after-bite prophylaxis with doxycycline most strongly indicated?
   a. A 6-year-old child resident in Connecticut from whom a fully *engorged dog tick* was removed yesterday
   b. A 55 year-old male resident of Louisiana from whom a slightly engorged adult Lone Star tick was removed yesterday
   c. An adult female patient resident in Connecticut from whom an engorged black-legged tick was removed 10 days ago
   d. An adult male resident of Rhode Island from whom a slightly engorged black-legged tick was removed yesterday
5. Which of the following methods are available to the public to reduce risk from Lyme disease in the environment?
   a. Vaccinating rodents
   b. Area-wide spraying with tick-killing products
   c. Pesticide treatment of deer
   d. Removal of wild animal reservoirs

Answers
   Answer 1: b
   Answer 2: b
   Answer 3: d
   Answer 4: d
   Answer 5: b

ACKNOWLEDGMENTS

The Pest Management Advisory Committee of the Department of National Defence provided an unpublished assessment on the efficacy of picaridin as a tick (and mosquito) repellent. Instructive comments and review of this article were kindly provided by Dr Ben Beard, CDC, Fort Collins.

REFERENCES

1. Centers for Disease Control and Prevention (CDC). Ticks geographic distribution. Available at: http://www.cdc.gov/ticks/geographic_distribution.html#blacklegged. Accessed April 27, 2015.
2. Public Health Agency of Canada. Established tick populations in Canada. Available at: http://www.phac-aspc.gc.ca/id-mi/tickinfo-eng.php. Accessed April 27, 2015.
3. Centers for Disease Control and Prevention (CDC). Lyme disease—data and statistics. Available at: http://www.cdc.gov/lyme/stats/. Accessed April 27, 2015.
4. Public Health Agency of Canada. National Lyme Disease Surveillance in Canada 2009–2012. Available at: http://healthycanadians.gc.ca/diseases-conditions-maladies-affections/disease-maladie/lyme/report-rapport-2009-2012-eng.php. Accessed April 27, 2015.
5. Stromdahl EY, Hickling GJ. Beyond Lyme: aetiology of tick-borne human diseases with emphasis on the south-eastern United States. Zoonoses Public Health 2012;59(Suppl 2):48–64.
6. Leighton PA, Koffi JK, Pelcat Y, et al. Predicting the speed of tick invasion: an empirical model of range expansion for the Lyme disease vector Ixodes scapularis in Canada. J Appl Ecol 2012;49(2):457–64.

7. Ogden NH, Lindsay LR, Leighton PA. Predicting the rate of invasion of the agent of Lyme disease Borrelia burgdorferi. J Appl Ecol 2013;50(2):510–8.

8. Poland GA. Vaccines against Lyme disease: what happened and what lessons can we learn? Clin Infect Dis 2011;52(Suppl 3):s253–8.

9. Hayes EB, Maupin GO, Mount GA, et al. Assessing the prevention effectiveness of local Lyme disease control. J Public Health Manag Pract 1999;5(3):84–92.

10. Poland GA. Prevention of Lyme disease: a review of the evidence. Mayo Clin Proc 2001;76(7):713–24.

11. Corapi KM, White MI, Phillips CB, et al. Strategies for primary and secondary prevention of Lyme disease. Nat Clin Pract Rheumatol 2007;3(1):20–5.

12. Piesman J, Eisen L. Prevention of tick-borne diseases. Annu Rev Entomol 2008; 53:323–43.

13. Piesman J, Beard CB. Prevention of tick-borne diseases. J Environ Health 2012; 74(10):30–2.

14. Ogden NH, Trudel L, Artsob H, et al. Ixodes scapularis ticks collected by passive surveillance in Canada: analysis of geographic distribution and infection with Lyme borreliosis agent Borrelia burgdorferi. J Med Entomol 2006;43(3): 600–9.

15. Ogden NH, Lindsay LR, Morshed M, et al. The emergence of Lyme disease in Canada. CMAJ 2009;180(12):1221–4.

16. Ogden NH, Koffi JK, Pelcat Y, et al. Environmental risk from Lyme disease in central and eastern Canada: a summary of recent surveillance information. Can Commun Dis Rep 2014;40(5):74–82.

17. Lindsay LR, Mathison SW, Barker IK, et al. Microclimate and habitat in relation to Ixodes scapularis (Acari: Ixodidae) populations on Long Point, Ontario, Canada. J Med Entomol 1999;36(3):255–62.

18. Guerra M, Walker E, Jones C, et al. Predicting the risk of Lyme disease: habitat suitability for Ixodes scapularis in the north central United States. Emerg Infect Dis 2002;8(3):289–97.

19. Smith RP. Ticks: the vectors of Lyme disease. In: Halperin JJ, editor. Lyme disease: an evidence based approach. Wallingford (CT); Oxfordshire (United Kingdom): CABI; 2011. p. 1–28.

20. Maupin GO, Fish D, Zultowsky J, et al. Landscape ecology of Lyme disease in a residential area of Westchester County, New York. Am J Epidemiol 1991; 133(11):1105–13.

21. Carroll MC, Ginsberg HS, Hyland KE, et al. Distribution of Ixodes dammini (Acari: Ixodidae) in residential lawns on Prudence Island, Rhode Island. J Med Entomol 1992;29(6):1052–5.

22. Duffy DC, Clark DD, Campbell SR, et al. Landscape patterns of abundance of Ixodes scapularis (Acari: Ixodidae) on Shelter Island, New York. J Med Entomol 1994;31(6):875–9.

23. Piesman J, Humair P. The spirochetes and vector ticks of Lyme borreliosis in nature. In: Sood SK, editor. Lyme Borreliosis in Europe and North America: epidemiology and clinical practice. Hoboken (NJ): John Wiley & Sons, Inc; 2011. p. 37–51.

24. Diuk-Wasser MA, Hoen AG, Cislo P, et al. Human risk of infection with Borrelia burgdorferi, the Lyme disease agent, in eastern United States. Am J Trop Med Hyg 2012;86(2):320–7.

25. Eisen RJ, Piesman J, Zielinski-Gutierrez E, et al. What do we need to know about disease ecology to prevent Lyme disease in the northeastern United States? J Med Entomol 2012;49(1):11–22.

26. Ogden NH, Lindsay LR, Hanincová K, et al. Role of migratory birds in introduction and range expansion of Ixodes scapularis ticks and of Borrelia burgdorferi and Anaplasma phagocytophilum in Canada. Appl Environ Microbiol 2008; 74(6):1780–90.

27. Rodgers SE, Miller NJ, Mather TN. Seasonal variation in nymphal blacklegged tick abundance in southern New England forests. J Med Entomol 2007;44(5):898–900.

28. Bacon RM, Kugeler KJ, Mead PS, et al. Surveillance for Lyme disease–United States, 1992–2006. MMWR Surveill Summ 2008;57(10):1–9.

29. Falco RC, Fish D, Piesman J. Duration of tick bites in a Lyme disease-endemic area. Am J Epidemiol 1996;143(2):187–92.

30. Clark RP, Hu LT. Prevention of Lyme disease and other tick-borne infections. Infect Dis Clin North Am 2008;22(3):381–96.

31. Duffy DC, Campbell SR. Ambient air temperature as a predictor of activity of adult Ixodes scapularis (Acari: Ixodidae). J Med Entomol 1994;31(1):178–80.

32. Vázquez M, Muehlenbein C, Cartter M, et al. Effectiveness of personal protective measures to prevent Lyme disease. Emerg Infect Dis 2008;14(2):210–6.

33. Schofield S, Plourde P. Statement on personal protective measures to prevent arthropod bites. An Advisory Committee Statement (ACS). Can Commun Dis Rep 2012;38(ACS-3):1–18.

34. Centers for Disease Control and Prevention (CDC). Preventing tick bites. Available at: http://www.cdc.gov/lyme/prev/index.html. Accessed April 27, 2015.

35. Health Canada. Pest Management Regulatory Agency. Insect Repellents. Available at: http://www.healthycanadians.gc.ca/environment-environnement/pesticides/insect_repellents-insectifuges-eng.php. Accessed April 27, 2015.

36. Health Canada. Pest Management Regulatory Agency. ARCHIVED - Memo - DEET (N,N-diethyl-m-toluamide) Statement of Guarantee and Labelling Allowances. Available at: http://www.hc-sc.gc.ca/cps-spc/pest/registrant-titulaire/prod/_memo-note/deet-eng.php. Accessed April 27, 2015.

37. Carroll SP. Prolonged efficacy of IR3535 repellents against mosquitoes and blacklegged ticks in North America. J Med Entomol 2008;45(4):706–14.

38. Cisak E, Wojcik-Fatla A, Zajac V, et al. Repellents and acaricides as personal protection measures in the prevention of tick-borne diseases. Ann Agric Environ Med 2012;19(4):625–30.

39. Pages F, Dautel H, Duvallet G, et al. Tick repellents for human use: prevention of tick bites and tick-borne diseases. Vector Borne Zoonotic Dis 2014;14(2):85–93.

40. Carroll JF, Kramer M. Different activities and footwear influence exposure to host-seeking nymphs of Ixodes scapularis and Amblyomma americanum (Acari: Ixodidae). J Med Entomol 2001;38(4):596–600.

41. Stjernberg L, Berglund J. Detecting ticks on light versus dark clothing. Scand J Infect Dis 2005;37(5):361–4.

42. Carroll JF. A cautionary note: survival of nymphs of two species of ticks (Acari: Ixodidae) among clothes laundered in an automatic washer. J Med Entomol 2003;40(5):732–6.

43. Evans SR, Korch GW Jr, Lawson MA. Comparative field evaluation of permethrin and DEET-treated military uniforms for personal protection against ticks (Acari). J Med Entomol 1990;27(5):829–34.

44. Miller NJ, Rainone EE, Dyer MC, et al. Tick bite protection with permethrin-treated summer-weight clothing. J Med Entomol 2011;48(2):327–33.

45. Vaughn MF, Meshnick SR. Pilot study assessing the effectiveness of long-lasting permethrin-impregnated clothing for the prevention of tick bites. Vector Borne Zoonotic Dis 2011;11(7):869–75.

46. Faulde MK, Rutenfranz M, Keth A, et al. Pilot study assessing the effectiveness of factory-treated, long-lasting permethrin-impregnated clothing for the prevention of tick bites during occupational tick exposure in highly infested military training areas, Germany. Parasitol Res 2015;114(2):671–8.

47. Vaughn MF, Funkhouser SW, Lin FC, et al. Long-lasting permethrin impregnated uniforms: a randomized-controlled trial for tick bite prevention. Am J Prev Med 2014;46(5):473–80.

48. Nasci RS, Zielinski-Gutierrez E, Wirtz RA, et al. CDC Yellow Book: Chapter 2—Protection against mosquitoes, ticks and other insects and arthropods. Available at: http://wwwnc.cdc.gov/travel/yellowbook/2014/chapter-2-the-pre-travel-consultation/protection-against-mosquitoes-ticks-and-other-insects-and-arthropods. Accessed April 27, 2015.

49. Connally NP, Durante AJ, Yousey-Hindes KM, et al. Peridomestic Lyme disease prevention. Results of a population-based case-control study. Am J Prev Med 2009;37(3):201–6.

50. Nadelman RB, Nowakowski J, Fish D, et al. Prophylaxis with single-dose doxycycline for the prevention of Lyme disease after an Ixodes scapularis tick bite. N Engl J Med 2001;345(2):79–84.

51. Mowbray F, Amlot R, Rubin GJ. Predictors of protective behaviour against ticks in the UK: a mixed methods study. Ticks Tick Borne Dis 2014;5(4): 392–400.

52. Needham GR. Evaluation of five popular methods for tick removal. Pediatrics 1985;75(6):997–1002.

53. Piesman J, Dolan MC. Protection against Lyme disease spirochete transmission provided by prompt removal of nymphal Ixodes scapularis (Acari: Ixodidae). J Med Entomol 2002;39(3):509–12.

54. Sood SK. Prevention of Lyme borreliosis. In: Sood SK, editor. Lyme borreliosis in Europe and North America: epidemiology and clinical practice. Hoboken (NJ): John Wiley & Sons, Inc; 2011. p. 225–44.

55. Duscher GG, Peschke R, Tichy A. Mechanical tools for the removal of Ixodes ricinus female ticks–differences of instruments and pulling or twisting? Parasitol Res 2012;111(4):1505–11.

56. Herrington JE Jr. Risk perceptions regarding ticks and Lyme disease: a national survey. Am J Prev Med 2004;26(2):135–40.

57. Gould LH, Nelson RS, Griffith KS, et al. Knowledge, attitudes, and behaviors regarding Lyme disease prevention among Connecticut residents, 1999–2004. Vector Borne Zoonotic Dis 2008;8(6):769–76.

58. Schofield S, Crane F, Tepper M. Good interventions that few use: uptake of insect bite precautions in a group of Canadian forces personnel deployed to Kabul, Afghanistan. Mil Med 2012;177(2):209–15.

59. Bayles BR, Evans G, Allan BF. Knowledge and prevention of tick-borne diseases vary across an urban-to-rural human land-use gradient. Ticks Tick Borne Dis 2013;4(4):352–8.

60. Hook SA, Nelson CA, Mead PS. U.S. public's experience with ticks and tick-borne diseases: results from national HealthStyles surveys. Ticks Tick Borne Dis 2015;6(4):483–8.

61. Stafford KC 3rd. Tick management handbook: an integrated guide for homeowners, pest control operators, and public health officials for the prevention of tick-associated disease. Bulletin 1010. New Haven (CT): Agricultural Experiment Station; 2007. p. 78.

62. Schulze TL, Jordan RA, Hung RW, et al. Efficacy of granular deltamethrin against Ixodes scapularis and Amblyomma americanum (Acari: Ixodidade) nymphs. J Med Entomol 2001;38(2):344–6.

63. Schulze TL, Jordan RA, Krivenko AJ. Effects of barrier application of granular deltamethrin on subadult Ixodes scapularis (Acari: Ixodidae) and nontarget forest floor arthropods. J Econ Entomol 2005;98(3):976–81.

64. Dolan MC, Jordan RA, Schulze TL, et al. Ability of two natural products, nootkatone and carvacrol, to suppress Ixodes scapularis and Amblyomma americanum (Acari: Ixodidae) in a Lyme disease endemic area of New Jersey. J Econ Entomol 2009;102(6):2316–24.

65. Rand PW, Lacombe EH, Elias SP, et al. Trial of a minimal-risk botanical compound to control the vector tick of Lyme disease. J Med Entomol 2010;47(4): 695–8.

66. Bharadwaj A, Stafford KC 3rd, Behle RW. Efficacy and environmental persistence of nootkatone for the control of the blacklegged tick (Acari: Ixodidae) in residential landscapes. J Med Entomol 2012;49(5):1035–44.

67. Kiss T, Cadar D, Spinu M. Tick prevention at a crossroad: new and renewed solutions. Vet Parasitol 2012;187(3–4):357–66.

68. Brei B, Brownstein JS, George JE, et al. Evaluation of the United States Department of Agriculture Northeast Area-wide Tick Control Project by meta-analysis. Vector Borne Zoonotic Dis 2009;9(4):423–30.

69. Dolan MC, Maupin GO, Schneider BS, et al. Control of immature Ixodes scapularis (Acari: Ixodidae) on rodent reservoirs of Borrelia burgdorferi in a residential community of southeastern Connecticut. J Med Entomol 2004;41(6): 1043–54.

70. Grear JS, Koethe R, Hoskins B, et al. The effectiveness of permethrin-treated deer stations for control of the Lyme disease vector Ixodes scapularis on Cape Cod and the islands: a five-year experiment. Parasit Vectors 2014;7:292.

71. Stafford KC 3rd, Kitron U. Environmental management for Lyme borreliosis control. In: Kahl O, Lane RS, Stanek G, editors. Lyme borreliosis biology, epidemiology and control. Wallingford (CT): CABI; 2002. p. 301–47.

72. Sorensen A, van Beest FM, Brook RK. Impacts of wildlife baiting and supplemental feeding on infectious disease transmission risk: a synthesis of knowledge. Prev Vet Med 2014;113(4):356–63.

73. Piesman J. Strategies for reducing the risk of Lyme borreliosis in North America. Int J Med Microbiol 2006;296(Suppl 40):17–22.

74. Wilson ML, Ducey AM, Litwin TS, et al. Microgeographic distribution of immature Ixodes dammini ticks correlated with that of deer. Med Vet Entomol 1990;4(2): 151–9.

75. Rand PW, Lubelczyk C, Lavigne GR, et al. Deer density and the abundance of Ixodes scapularis (Acari: Ixodidae). J Med Entomol 2003;40(2):179–84.

76. Jordan RA, Schulze TL, Jahn MB. Effects of reduced deer density on the abundance of Ixodes scapularis (Acari: Ixodidae) and Lyme disease incidence in a northern New Jersey endemic area. J Med Entomol 2007;44(5):752–7.

77. Kilpatrick HJ, LaBonte AM, Stafford KC. The relationship between deer density, tick abundance, and human cases of Lyme disease in a residential community. J Med Entomol 2014;51(4):777–84.

78. Rand PW, Lubelczyk C, Holman MS, et al. Abundance of Ixodes scapularis (Acari: Ixodidae) after the complete removal of deer from an isolated offshore island, endemic for Lyme disease. J Med Entomol 2004;41(4):779–84.

79. McShea WJ. Ecology and management of white-tailed deer in a changing world. Ann N Y Acad Sci 2012;1249:45–56.

80. In Defense of Animals. Anti-Hunting. Available at: http://www.idausa.org/campaigns/wild-free2/habitats-campaign/anti-hunting/. Accessed April 27, 2015.

81. Stafford KC 3rd. Reduced abundance of Ixodes scapularis (Acari: Ixodidae) with exclusion of deer by electric fencing. J Med Entomol 1993;30(6):986–96.

82. Daniels TJ, Fish D. Effect of deer exclusion on the abundance of immature Ixodes scapularis (Acari: Ixodidae) parasitizing small and medium-sized mammals. J Med Entomol 1995;32(1):5–11.

83. Del Fabbro S. Fencing and mowing as effective methods for reducing tick abundance on very small, infested plots. Ticks Tick Borne Dis 2015;6(2):167–72.

84. Ley C, Olshen EM, Reingold AL. Case-control study of risk factors for incident Lyme disease in California. Am J Epidemiol 1995;142(9 Suppl):S39–47.

85. Goossens HA, van den Bogaard AE, Nohlmans MK. Dogs as sentinels for human Lyme borreliosis in The Netherlands. J Clin Microbiol 2001;39(3):844–8.

86. Berrada ZL, Telford SR 3rd. Burden of tick-borne infections on American companion animals. Top Companion Anim Med 2009;24(4):175–81.

87. Rabinowitz PM, Gordon Z, Odofin L. Pet-related infections. Am Fam Physician 2007;76(9):1314–22.

88. Richer LM, Brisson D, Melo R, et al. Reservoir targeted vaccine against Borrelia burgdorferi: a new strategy to prevent Lyme disease transmission. J Infect Dis 2014;209(12):1972–80.

89. Gomes-Solecki M. Blocking pathogen transmission at the source: reservoir targeted OspA-based vaccines against Borrelia burgdorferi. Front Cell Infect Microbiol 2014;4:136.

90. Tsao JI, Wootton JT, Bunikis J, et al. An ecological approach to preventing human infection: vaccinating wild mouse reservoirs intervenes in the Lyme disease cycle. Proc Natl Acad Sci U S A 2004;101(52):18159–64.

91. Tsao K, Fish D, Galvani AP. Predicted outcomes of vaccinating wildlife to reduce human risk of Lyme disease. Vector Borne Zoonotic Dis 2012;12(7):544–51.

92. Berger KA, Ginsberg HS, Dugas KD, et al. Adverse moisture events predict seasonal abundance of Lyme disease vector ticks (Ixodes scapularis). Parasit Vectors 2014;7:181.

93. Wilson ML. Reduced abundance of adult Ixodes dammini (Acari: Ixodidae) following destruction of vegetation. J Econ Entomol 1986;79(3):693–6.

94. Schulze TL, Jordan RA, Hung RW. Suppression of subadult Ixodes scapularis (Acari: Ixodidae) following removal of leaf litter. J Med Entomol 1995;32(5):730–3.

95. Mather TN, Duffy DC, Campbell SR. An unexpected result from burning vegetation to reduce Lyme disease transmission risks. J Med Entomol 1993;30(3):642–5.

96. Stafford KC 3rd, Ward JS, Magnarelli LA. Impact of controlled burns on the abundance of Ixodes scapularis (Acari: Ixodidae). J Med Entomol 1998;35(4):510–3.

97. Williams SC, Ward JS. Effects of Japanese barberry (Ranunculales: Berberidaceae) removal and resulting microclimatic changes on Ixodes scapularis (Acari: Ixodidae) abundances in Connecticut, USA. Environ Entomol 2010;39(6):1911–21.

98. Stafford KC 3rd, Allan SA. Field applications of entomopathogenic fungi Beauveria bassiana and Metarhizium anisopliae F52 (Hypocreales: Clavicipitaceae)

for the control of Ixodes scapularis (Acari: Ixodidae). J Med Entomol 2010;47(6): 1107–15.

99. Bharadwaj A, Stafford KC 3rd. Evaluation of Metarhizium anisopliae strain F52 (Hypocreales: Clavicipitaceae) for control of Ixodes scapularis (Acari: Ixodidae). J Med Entomol 2010;47(5):862–7.

100. Fernandes EK, Bittencourt VR, Roberts DW. Perspectives on the potential of entomopathogenic fungi in biological control of ticks. Exp Parasitol 2012;130(3): 300–5.

101. Duffy DC, Downer R, Brinkley C. The effectiveness of Helmeted Guneafowl in the control of the deer tick, the vector of Lyme disease. Wilson Bulletin 1992; 104:342.

102. Hinckley A, Meek J, Ray J, et al. Efficacy of a single peridomestic application of acaricide to prevent Lyme and other tick-borne diseases. Presented at: 13th International Conference on Lyme Borreliosis and Other Tick-Borne Diseases. Boston (MA), August 18–21, 2013.

103. Nigrovic LE, Thompson KM. The Lyme vaccine: a cautionary tale. Epidemiol Infect 2007;135(1):1–8.

104. Marconi RT, Earnhart CG. Lyme disease vaccines. In: Samuels DS, Radolf JD, editors. Borrelia: molecular biology, host interaction and pathogenesis. Norfolk (United Kingdom): Caister Academic Press; 2010. p. 467–86.

105. Costello CM, Steere AC, Pinkerton RE, et al. A prospective study of tick bites in an endemic area for Lyme disease. J Infect Dis 1989;159(1):136–9.

106. Shapiro ED, Gerber MA, Holabird NB, et al. A controlled trial of antimicrobial prophylaxis for Lyme disease after deer-tick bites. N Engl J Med 1992; 327(25):1769–73.

107. Agre F, Schwartz R. The value of early treatment of deer tick bites for the prevention of Lyme disease. Am J Dis Child 1993;147(9):945–7.

108. Warshafsky S, Lee DH, Francois LK, et al. Efficacy of antibiotic prophylaxis for the prevention of Lyme disease: an updated systematic review and meta-analysis. J Antimicrob Chemother 2010;65(6):1137–44.

109. Wormser GP, Dattwyler RJ, Shapiro ED, et al. The clinical assessment, treatment, and prevention of Lyme disease, human granulocytic anaplasmosis, and babesiosis: clinical practice guidelines by the Infectious Diseases Society of America. Clin Infect Dis 2006;43(9):1089–134.

110. Institute of Medicine. Clinical Practice Guidelines We Can Trust. Washington, DC: The National Academies Press; 2011.

111. Perea AE, Hinckley AF, Mead PS. Tick bite prophylaxis: results from a 2012 survey of healthcare providers. Zoonoses Public Health 2015;62(5):388–92.

112. Brett ME, Hinckley AF, Zielinski-Gutierrez EC, et al. U.S. healthcare providers' experience with Lyme and other tick-borne diseases. Ticks Tick Borne Dis 2014;5(4):404–8.

113. Bissinger BW, Roe RM. Tick repellents: past, present, and future. Pestic Biochem Physiol 2010;96(2):63–79.

114. Katz TM, Miller JH, Hebert AA. Insect repellents: historical perspectives and new developments. J Am Acad Dermatol 2008;58(5):865–71.

115. Shadick NA, Daltroy LH, Phillips CB, et al. Determinants of tick-avoidance behaviors in an endemic area for Lyme disease. Am J Prev Med 1997;13(4): 265–70.

United States Postal Service

Statement of Ownership, Management, and Circulation
(All Periodicals Publications Except Requestor Publications)

1. Publication Title	2. Publication Number	3. Filing Date
Clinics in Laboratory Medicine	0 1 2 - 9 6 0	9/18/15

4. Issue Frequency	5. Number of Issues Published Annually	6. Annual Subscription Price
Mar, Jun, Sep, Dec	4	$250.00

7. Complete Mailing Address of Known Office of Publication *(Not printer) (Street, city, county, state, and ZIP+4®)*

Elsevier Inc.
360 Park Avenue South
New York, NY 10010-1710

Contact Person
Stephen R. Bushing
Telephone: *(Include area code)*
215-239-3688

8. Complete Mailing Address of Headquarters or General Business Office of Publisher *(Not printer)*

Elsevier Inc., 360 Park Avenue South, New York, NY 10010-1710

9. Full Names and Complete Mailing Addresses of Publisher, Editor, and Managing Editor *(Do not leave blank)*

Publisher *(Name and complete mailing address)*

Linda Belfus, Elsevier Inc., 1600 John F. Kennedy Blvd., Suite 1800, Philadelphia, PA 19103

Editor *(Name and complete mailing address)*

Lauren Boyle, Elsevier Inc., 1600 John F. Kennedy Blvd., Suite 1800, Philadelphia, PA 19103-2899

Managing Editor *(Name and complete mailing address)*

Adrianne Brigido, Elsevier Inc., 1600 John F. Kennedy Blvd., Suite 1800, Philadelphia, PA 19103-2899

10. Owner *(Do not leave blank. If the publication is owned by a corporation, give the name and address of the corporation immediately followed by the names and addresses of all stockholders owning or holding 1 percent or more of the total amount of stock. If not owned by a corporation, give the names and addresses of the individual owners. If owned by a partnership or other unincorporated firm, give its name and address as well as those of each individual owner. If the publication is published by a nonprofit organization, give its name and address.)*

Full Name	Complete Mailing Address
Wholly owned subsidiary of	1600 John F. Kennedy Blvd. Ste. 1800
Reed/Elsevier, US holdings	Philadelphia, PA 19103-2899

11. Known Bondholders, Mortgagees, and Other Security Holders Owning or Holding 1 Percent or More of Total Amount of Bonds, Mortgages, or Other Securities. If none, check box. ▸ ☐ None

Full Name	Complete Mailing Address
N/A	

12. Tax Status *(For completion by nonprofit organizations authorized to mail at nonprofit rates) (Check one)*
The purpose, function, and nonprofit status of this organization and the exempt status for federal income tax purposes:
☐ Has Not Changed During Preceding 12 Months
☐ Has Changed During Preceding 12 Months *(Publisher must submit explanation of change with this statement)*

PS Form 3526, July 2014 [Page 1 of 3 (Instructions Page 3)] PSN 7530-01-000-9931 PRIVACY NOTICE: See our Privacy policy in www.usps.com

---

13. Publication Title	14. Issue Date for Circulation Data Below
Clinics in Laboratory Medicine	September 2015

15. Extent and Nature of Circulation			Average No. Copies Each Issue During Preceding 12 Months	No. Copies of Single Issue Published Nearest to Filing Date
a. Total Number of Copies *(Net press run)*			200	268
b. Legitimate Paid and/or Requested Distribution *(By Mail and Outside the Mail)*	(1)	Market Outside County Paid/Requested Mail Subscriptions stated on PS Form 3541. *(Include paid distribution above nominal rate, advertiser's proof copies and exchange copies)*	83	70
	(2)	Mailed In-County Paid/Requested Mail Subscriptions stated on PS Form 3541. *(Include paid distribution above nominal rate, advertiser's proof copies and exchange copies)*	46	55
	(3)	Paid Distribution Outside the Mails Including Sales Through Dealers And Carriers, Street Vendors, Counter Sales, and Other Paid Distribution Outside USPS®		
	(4)	Paid Distribution by Other Classes of Mail Through the USPS (e.g. First-Class Mail®)		
c. Total Paid and or Requested Circulation *(Sum of 15b (1), (2), (3), and (4))* ▸			129	125
d. Free or Nominal Rate Distribution *(By Mail and Outside the Mail)*	(1)	Free or Nominal Rate Outside-County Copies included on PS Form 3541	63	62
	(2)	Free or Nominal Rate In-County Copies included on PS Form 3541		
	(3)	Free or Nominal Rate Copies mailed at Other classes Through the USPS (e.g. First-Class Mail®)		
	(4)	Free or Nominal Rate Distribution Outside the Mail *(Carriers or Other means)*		
e. Total Nonrequested Distribution *(Sum of 15d (1), (2), (3) and (4))* ▸			63	62
f. Total Distribution *(Sum of 15c and 15e)* ▸			192	187
g. Copies not Distributed *(See instructions to publishers #4 (page #3))* ▸			8	81
h. Total *(Sum of 15f and g)* ▸			200	268
i. Percent Paid and/or Requested Circulation *(15c divided by 15f times 100)* ▸			67.19%	66.84%

* If you are claiming electronic copies go to line 16 on page 3. If you are not claiming Electronic copies, skip to line 17 on page 3.

16. Electronic Copy Circulation	Average No. Copies Each Issue During Preceding 12 Months	No. Copies of Single Issue Published Nearest to Filing Date
a. Paid Electronic Copies ▸		
b. Total paid Print Copies (Line 15c) + Paid Electronic copies (Line 16a) ▸		
c. Total Print Distribution (Line 15f) + Paid Electronic Copies (Line 16a) ▸		
d. Percent Paid (Both Print & Electronic copies) (16b divided by 16c X 100) ▸		

☐ I certify that 50% of all my distributed copies (electronic and print) are paid above a nominal price.

17. Publication of Statement of Ownership
☒ If the publication is a general publication, publication of this statement is required. Will be printed in the **December 2015** issue of this publication.

18. Signature and Title of Editor, Publisher, Business Manager, or Owner   Date

Stephen R. Bushing
Stephen R. Bushing – Inventory Distribution Coordinator   September 18, 2015

I certify that all information furnished on this form is true and complete. I understand that anyone who furnishes false or misleading information on this form or who omits material or information requested on the form may be subject to criminal sanctions (including fines and imprisonment) and/or civil sanctions (including civil penalties).

PS Form 3526, July 2014 (Page 3 of 3)

Moving?

Make sure your subscription moves with you!

To notify us of your new address, find your **Clinics Account Number** (located on your mailing label above your name), and contact customer service at:

Email: journalscustomerservice-usa@elsevier.com

800-654-2452 (subscribers in the U.S. & Canada)
314-447-8871 (subscribers outside of the U.S. & Canada)

Fax number: 314-447-8029

Elsevier Health Sciences Division
Subscription Customer Service
3251 Riverport Lane
Maryland Heights, MO 63043

Printed and bound by CPI Group (UK) Ltd, Croydon, CR0 4YY

03/10/2024

01040491-0019